Maria del rosario Angeles
Sarai Morales

"Guide for the correct accompaniment in sphincter control."

Maria del rosario Angeles
Sarai Morales

"Guide for the correct accompaniment in sphincter control."

"Guide for the correct accompaniment in sphincter control in children from 18 months to 3 years of age."

ScienciaScripts

Imprint
Any brand names and product names mentioned in this book are subject to trademark, brand or patent protection and are trademarks or registered trademarks of their respective holders. The use of brand names, product names, common names, trade names, product descriptions etc. even without a particular marking in this work is in no way to be construed to mean that such names may be regarded as unrestricted in respect of trademark and brand protection legislation and could thus be used by anyone.

Cover image: www.ingimage.com

This book is a translation from the original published under ISBN 978-620-2-24079-6.

Publisher:
Sciencia Scripts
is a trademark of
Dodo Books Indian Ocean Ltd. and OmniScriptum S.R.L Publishing group
Str. Armeneasca 28/1, office 1, Chisinau-2012, Republic of Moldova, Europe
Printed at: see last page
ISBN: 978-620-5-25935-1

Copyright © Maria del rosario Angeles, Sarai Morales
Copyright © 2022 Dodo Books Indian Ocean Ltd. and OmniScriptum S.R.L Publishing group

"GUIDE FOR THE CORRECT ACCOMPANIMENT IN SPHINCTER CONTROL IN CHILDREN FROM 18 MONTHS TO 3 YEARS OF AGE".

INTRODUCTION

The interest of this research is directed to a latent problem in the development of the infant, sphincter control is already a natural process that happens in the human body and development, it is important to emphasize that in the investigation of sphincter control several arguments are known about what it entails, how to carry it and the success behind; the idea is focused on being a support for parents and teachers, since it is known about the subject, but it is often used wrongly making this a problematic and negative process.Likewise, sphincter control conflicts lead to serious health problems and most of the time they are unknown by parents, because they only think that if they leave the diaper on longer nothing will happen, without recognizing that there are consequences, as well as knowing that development takes into account the growth and improvement of functional skills, It is incredible to know that a correct neurological development helps to control the sphincter and that the sphincter is a muscle that must be well developed to be able to work it, as well as to understand that nighttime sphincter control takes longer to mature.The pillar of the research is child care in order to support the good emotional development of the child, recognizing the capacity of this, knowing that it can be accompanied successfully, having positive results first at home both in kindergarten or school, being a support in The research emphasizes how toilet training can go from being something natural and progressive, with enough signals from the body to initiate it, to a process that is harmful to the infant's emotional and physical health.The development of sphincter control serves the child to be a path to independence, as it gives the ability of self-control, the fact of a good accompaniment will result in confident and independent children or children full of doubt, shame and fear, it is very important to recognize how the support and encouragement of parents and teachers together will give good or bad results.The work will be based on children from 18 months to 3 years of age who are beginning with sphincter control, which have specific characteristics according to the stage of development in which they find themselves.

Problem statement:

In the 18 months to 3 years stage, children experience a series of physiological changes that will help control their sphincters, which is a key point in their development. Unfortunately, different situations have caused repercussions in this stage.Beginning to experience the physiological changes, the stages of attachment, facing heavy grooming burdens, makes this process often drags on looking for the easiest way out or solution without realizing that this is detrimental to a child.Since it involves everything from emotional problems to health problems, this stage is no different in kindergartens or preschools, where it is a not very positive experience for both teachers and students.The child who is in the process becomes a burden and often suffers the consequences of stress and despair, since there is no empathy to support or understand this succession to the extent of duping emotions and feelings.

The problem lies in seeing the consequences of such actions to hasten the process or lengthen it such as: low self-esteem, fear, tantrums, regression, etc. And recognize that potty training problems are often based on moments that can cause trauma or unpleasantness for children.

Research question

A correct accompaniment in the development of the sphincter control allows to promote a better learning of the same, shorter and more concrete, so it will allow him to conclude it in a shorter time without damaging his integrity, therefore:
How to support parents and teachers with the process of toilet training?

Hypothesis

The creation of an accompanying guide for children from 18 months to 3 years of age will favor total mastery of sphincter control.

General Objective

To create a guide for a correct accompaniment of sphincter control in support of parents, family, tutors and teachers, raising awareness of the importance of the child's maturation.

Specific objective

To disseminate information on the correct accompaniment of the child in toilet training and the benefits of doing it in a positive way.

Justification

Children aged 18 months to 3 years in the biological process of toilet training are already fully developed in the sensory-motor scheme because they already perceive the world through their senses, as they begin to develop different skills, we are talking about a neurological maturation in which they acquire achievements in their autonomy, since the development of their gross and fine motor skills and toilet training will produce pleasure in the infant. It will focus on determining the situation that parents and children live in the beginning of the sphincter control and how a poorly guided process totally affects the infant, altering different natural processes, creating insecurities, affecting their self-esteem, etc.

General Description

The motivation to investigate the effects of poor potty training is based on the fact that it is clearly known that it has had serious effects on this sector of the population. exposed and is more vulnerable than the rest, strengthening the risks involved. We intend, then, to help alert about this danger and the damage to the child's self-esteem, health and development, as well as to generate knowledge that will help in the process and control the effects produced by ignorance and tension. In this research we can find key points for toilet training, the characteristics of the child's maturation and most importantly, a guide created especially for parents and teachers so that they can take the process hand in hand, making it easier for both without letting one do more and miss the advanced and most importantly to have fundamentals of what is being used.

CHAPTER 1

STAGES OF CHILD DEVELOPMENT

All the older people were, at first, children, although few of them remember it.
--Antoine de Saint-Exupéry

In this chapter we will talk about the development of the child, as we already know the development starts from conception, early childhood, infancy, puberty, adolescence, adulthood, where we can know the processes by which there are different changes, some notorious, some not so much, but equally important, to know the path that the body takes to demonstrate the changes it needs and make the body functional, determine that the growth and development does not stop or reorganize but it works in a natural way.We will recognize the stages of development in depth and know the processes involved, in the same way we will learn about emotional development and how it is linked to toilet training, what is toilet training in a clearer way, parenting styles, differences and how they influence toilet training.This will be done mainly to support parents, because we know that the beginning of all development is mainly at home and we will emphasize the need to support the infant emotionally in order to not emotionally damaging and disruptive to the process of toilet training. First we will address the stages of child development and learn how they relate to toilet training.

1.1 Stages of development

The stages of child development encompass the physical, emotional and social. Social development is known to be the place where the child develops, the theories of the stages of child development divide it in different ways, also taking into account the society in which the child develops. For example, in some it is divided into three stages, infancy, childhood, and adult life; others only in two childhoods and adult life; the society in which the child develops will determine which stages he will experience, therefore, this will influence his development, we see it according to Hoffmann "The way in which individuals in a society contemplate the life cycle depends largely on its social and economic system, for example during the Middle Ages childhood lasted until 7 years" (Craig, et al., 1996).Each phase of the child has its own characteristics, which when developed correctly will determine if the child grows up to be a happy and fulfilled adult in every sense; the physical changes of each stage are very noticeable; they include from the fall of teeth, growth, weight gain, to hair growth in adolescence; as for the psychological growth, this goes hand in hand with the physical by relating the child's growth and its relationship with the world around it, using its experiences from the stage of its birth to change the perception it has of the environment. Growth is undoubtedly something inevitable that happens to every human being, the important thing is to recognize the changes; of utmost importance for teachers, but fundamental for parents; recognizing and knowing how to support the child in this natural development that the body and thought undergoes should make it a pillar in the life of parents.The author of the psychosexual theory Sigmund Freud divides child development into stages in which the child develops a response to stimuli, either in personality, character, physical, etc..This theory is still very controversial, as it touches sensitive issues today and understands that children's impulses are released or focused on erogenous zones and through certain attitudes and stages they experience it as a consequence; the development is focused on understanding why these are linked to sphincter control, since there is a specific stage in the theory of psychoanalysis mentioned by the author Sigmund Freud that focuses specifically on the subject, according to Font we can see that:The second of these phases is the ANAL PHASE, which lasts from the first year and a half until the age of three. In this phase, sensitivity will be directed to the anal mucosa and the act of defecation - without forgetting oral pleasure - which will appear as a new focus of pleasurable sensations, reinforced by the learning of sphincter control. This learning will lead to the appearance of the first prohibitions, and also of the first 'gifts' (feces). In parallel with the pleasure that the child obtains through defecation, there is the reality of cleanliness, and the control to which this is subjected by the environment. The child learns that it produces something valuable and that his control allows him, to a certain extent, to manipulate his mother (Font, 1990 p.4).It can be recognized that the second phase of the theory of psychoanalysis is closely linked to sphincter control, remember that the process of sphincter control occurs during the stage that Freud named "anal phase", taking into account that the act of defecation takes a very important role for the sensitivity of the infant and as the succession to cleaning makes him feel pleasure in its development.It also establishes a new form of relationship that can be experienced as something beneficial (cleanliness) and satisfactory (the mother's joy) or as an imposition that is difficult to accept. It is also possible to observe games with feces or with substitutes (sand, mud, etc.). It is a stage in which a certain process of autonomy and self-affirmation begins.At this stage, the need to explore the body will also begin to manifest itself with intensity, which will make him contact his genital organs that he will manipulate to obtain pleasure (in the following stage this need will be even greater) (Font, 1990 p.4).As it can be read, the process can be satisfactory or taken as a demand and it is reaffirmed that in this period an atmosphere of good, independence or the opposite of heteronomy is created, so that self-exploration begins and therefore the discovery of oneself and different sensations. The author Erik Erikson impacts the social environment, with the development of his theory of psychosocial stages reconstructed on the basis of Freud's psychosexual theory, which cover the complete development of the person and are:Trust versus distrust stage, where the author touches on how the child in the stage from 0 to 18 months will have a change in his personality, taking into account if his basic needs such as food, care, love, affection are covered, this will influence his trust, of course every child must develop a certain degree of distrust to obtain care in dangerous situations, but this will be triggered if the child feels abandoned and isolated or loved and cared for.Stage, autonomy versus shame, which covers from 2 to 3 years, in this stage the author touches on the issue of retention and elimination, in addition to hygiene, and autonomy, in this stage we can focus on the issue of sphincter control, as the child will have the ability to feel shame which will help create a habit of retention until reaching the toilet; remember that the adult is responsible for not hurting psychologically so that the child can trust himself/herself.Stage, initiative versus guilt and fear, from 3 to 5 years of age, in which the child begins to show affection to third parties outside his family context, to demonstrate his own interests, begins to learn through play and roles in his imagination and to know how to separate fantasy from reality. In total, psychosocial theory speaks of 8 stages, but we will focus on the first three and mainly on the second stage, because the issue of sphincter control plays an important role and is developed in that stage.Another author who touches the subject of child development is Vigostky in the learning environment, a game made up of cognitive stages supported by Piaget in which we can know the evolution of thinking, knowledge, skills, understanding, on which the author emphasizes the social context of the child and how this has an effect on their development. The importance of the stages helps us to know in which biological and social development we are according to our maturity and lived process, that is why thanks to the knowledge of these stages we can know if a child is ready to start potty training or can wait a little to start it.

1.2 What is sphincter control.

To know the meaning of the process of sphincter control and to recognize the succession of cognitive processes involved in bladder and digestive tract control, which is medically called a hygiene process related to defecation and urination takes a succession during childhood and as it is known it is an acquired procedure because it involves certain physiological and cognitive maturation to achieve one hundred percent control. In most cases, the sequence in the acquisition of voluntary sphincter control begins with bowel control during sleep, followed by fecal control during waking hours, then daytime urine control, and finally nighttime control. Many children acquire bowel and bladder control simultaneously.
There are interindividual and intercultural variations, influenced by educational, family, social, psychological and hereditary factors (Garza, 2020, p.40).Remembering that urine control is carried out more quickly and concisely than stool control, which takes a little longer; also taking into account nighttime control, which evolves a little slower; the need for maturation is an important point along with the child's emotional abilities, neuromotor capacity, each point must be adapted to the child's needs in order to respect his learning pace, taking into account that everyone has different learning processes.As such, the sphincter is a muscle that certainly must be exercised to have a mastery of it, so carrying a well-stimulated accompaniment, constancy and respect will help to achieve the goal of this control; "Sphincter control is the result of a process that has comings and goings, it is not linear and admits, sloppiness, like any new learning that we try" (Ramirez & Rivera, 2015, p.3).Each child's learning process is carried out step by step, therefore, it is not achieved one hundred percent from one day to the next, in addition to a series of steps or situations that must be taken into account.Sphincter control is located in an age

range, which ranges from 2 to 3 years of age, but it is important to emphasize that it is not something strictly established, and since children who begin a process between one and a half and two years of age, require a cognitive maturation, as well as a guided and gradual accompaniment, it is counterproductive in some cases, since learning is taken gradually to be better established and there are no negative interferences;

Therefore, a relaxed environment, supported by parents, will result in a training that gives better results in less time.Bearing in mind that toilet training is something very important in the growth process of a child, therefore, it should not be underestimated and all parents should know what characteristics are involved in this process; toilet training is linked to prevent actions, so that controlling urine or defecation involves preventing them from being released at any time, therefore, the child reaches a brain maturity.As mentioned above, the process of sphincter control has characteristics that are quite involved as a maturity of the nervous system, this maturation makes the child able to recognize when the bladder is full, when he already has the need to urinate or defecate, is then when the signals begin to begin to guide children in their visits to the bathroom, something important would be to emphasize that the control will not be achieved if not taken into account the necessary maturity in the nervous system, from Likewise, recognize that it is not just any learning, but involves brain processes and maturity of the system.To achieve sphincter control requires the adequate acquisition of developmental milestones: that the child walks, understands and expresses himself verbally; that he has a good level of affective maturation, with development of anal and urethral tendencies, and that he has a family prepared and willing to accompany and guide the training process (Garza, 2020, p. 41).As we can see, it emphasizes once again the importance of the maturation of developmental milestones[1] and a family that is prepared together with the child to start this process in the best way and emphasizes that if we want to achieve a correct control, we must take into account what the child is already doing.In conclusion, toilet training should not begin before 18 months of age. After that age there is much variability in determining the appropriate time at which the child is ready for toilet training to begin. The parents' decision to initiate training should be based on the child's socioemotional and psychological maturity. Studies show that the earlier intensive toilet training begins, the younger the child will become, but the longer it will take for toilet training to begin. (Garza, 2020, p.42).Not forcing or pressuring the child will make his learning more autonomous, lighter and he will know how to cope with the difficulties, there are important points to consider on the part of the parents; to begin with, it is necessary not to be forced by age or by comments from outside the family, because many times the pressure of society makes the child fall into being pressured, even before the time he may achieve it, but later it will bring serious consequences in the child's development.There are many consequences when dealing with hasty sphincter control such as: frustration of the child and parents, fear of advancement or accidents, crying, low self-esteem, depression, insecurity, grief, and physical problems such as constipation, irritable or lazy colon, enuresis, encopresis, etc. That said, their socioemotional development must also be taken care of, since it will greatly influence their growth.

1.3 What is socioemotional development?

During childhood the child is predisposed to develop an emotional temperament due to the interaction he/she has with the environment, taking into account that the affectation of the emotional goes hand in hand with aspects of his/her life and family context such as economics, sex, relationship with parents, etc. The socioemotional development includes that the child will be able to develop his emotions well, recognizing them and taking into account his social relationship with his environment. Social-emotional development involves a series of steps in which the child becomes socially and emotionally competent in order to grow and develop fully as an adult. Emotional competencies are:Self-regulation should be developed in children so that they know how to react to negative situations such as tantrums, anger, frustration tolerance that will avoid bad moments and situations of anxiety for their age, because when faced with difficult situations they do not have enough control or lose it easily, so they must begin to have self-control because at their age it is not so easy to express ideas and needs because of their limited language and movement. Another emotional competence is the recognition and expression of their emotion, it consists of knowing what emotion they are feeling and recognizing the emotions of those around them, this should be categorized by naming their own and others' emotions.Social skills consist of knowing, developing empathy, examining the emotion of others and being able to regulate that emotion or help in the situation, and relating to others will help the child to understand his or her own needs and those of others.Autonomy in children is important, as it gives a boost to their own being, helps them to be self-sufficient, not depending on an adult to perform any task or activity, which are according to their age and development. An emotionally competent child will know how to regulate his emotions in a positive way to achieve progress without harming others, therefore, if a child manages to be socially competent, he will have the ability to engage and relate to friends, family, peers in a positive way.

The concept of socioemotional development includes the acquisition of a series of capacities, such as self-regulation and attention, the ability to establish relationships, social interactions, reciprocity, and social problem solving through the meaningful use of language, which occurs through a series of developmental milestones that are reached in the first 4 years of life. (Farkas & Rodriguez, 2017, p. 2736). In the first years of life, the child develops a series of characteristics that help him/her to develop correctly, such as self-confidence, therefore, several aptitudes are taken into account that will provide the child with autonomy, self-control and will make him/her socially open or sufficiently apt to show his/her decisions and emotions.A child learns to develop emotionally when he relates to himself, because he begins to recognize his emotions and to know how to express them; this will result in a positive impact in different areas of his life, such as the child's ability to learn and develop his skills. The family will be an important starting point, since it is the first context where the child begins his or her socioemotional development, the first place where knows what is right and what is wrong, thus triggering positive or problematic situations.Taking into account that the relationship mainly with the mother will determine the way in which the child develops socioemotionally, since if the child has a mother with a positive attachment pattern, the child will have better weapons and foundations when facing stressful and negative situations; considering that a better socioemotionally developed child is also affected by his economic context, since if he has a low economic stability, the stress and problems of the parents will notably affect the child, resulting in a child with low self-esteem, without knowing how to control emotions, poor temperament management, etc.At the age in which the child develops sphincter control, social and emotional development also plays a part, which, if guided by understanding and empathetic parents, the child will develop the ability to control emotions and be socially open, as he/she will no longer be afraid of new experiences and activities because he/she had enough support from the first context he/she met. It is extremely important to emphasize that a nurturing environment will result in fewer problems in early childhood development, which will have repercussions until adolescence. Not knowing how to recognize emotions and stressful experiences in the development process will drag the child through one of the most difficult ages for human beings.People with higher levels of socioemotional development present higher indicators of general well-being and less depressive symptoms, and greater satisfaction in their interpersonal relationships, recent studies show an association between socioemotional aspects and different academic indicators, such as performance, learning and content mastery, motivation and engagement (Berger, Milicic, Alcalay, & Torretti, 2014, p. 107).Socioemotional development not only has crucial effects in negative situations, but in the whole development, because it can be seen that a better growth will bring with it good aspects to fulfill that will help to be a better human being and a better person in all aspects. Therefore, socioemotional development has repercussions in all senses and it is relevant to take it into account in this research, because we can know how a good accompaniment in growth will help the optimal development of the child and will help in all developmental milestones. It is crucial as parents to have patience and support the development of our children, generating an environment of trust through the type of parenting established at home. In this case we are going to describe the positive parenting style and how it emotionally affects the development of the child's potty training.

1.4 Positive parenting style

Over time, parenting styles have been modified by generations, we know strict generations, where the parenting style was authoritarian, based on the control of parents or guardians, establishing rules and intimidating infants. As a result of this, children develop fear, insecurity of failure, low self-esteem and as a result we have adults lacking control of emotions with anxiety and other affectations. Moving on to a permissive parenting style, where parents who manage this parenting style were usually brought up with an authoritarian parenting style, where by means of the method used, they allow any action, they are unconcerned with toilet training, and let the child decide freely; as a consequence of this they let the child decide freely; as a consequence of this we can observe that the children have a delay in the control of sphincters, or a setback, as it is their decision, they do it anywhere, such as the playground, the corridors, since the motto of permissive parents is to have a free soul and let them be.Let's think about which parenting style is the right one, even if the generations of the 70's, 80's, 90's educated us with this type of authoritarian parenting styles, we can say that the current generations are the ones who are wrong, Actually the adults who are educating these children today are adults who were raised with this type of parenting styles, that is limited children, to explore, discover, analyze, but like all these children, some became leaders, generating new work expectations, we can say that the generations also have a great social impact, that is, this generation of authoritarian style, is the person you find in the street exploiting the children's rights, and that is the one you find in the street exploiting the children's rights. anger, frustration, anger, or people who have a hard time progressing, or people who are responsible, and are fulfilled at work, it is a great social paradigm to be able to observe the generations, from the form of education. Well moving on to another parenting style that is found in the formative generations of society is the permissive parenting style, observing the teaching ranges there are different theories where it is considered that adults who were limited, and harassed; by the authoritarian parenting style, having different traumas in childhood is why they tend not to want to follow patterns of education, making the mistake of leaving or allowing any behavior.This is also confusing, we see extremes of education or parenting style, so we reached a stage or era where generations are concerned about understanding each of the cognitive processes or stages of infants, positive parenting style, where the foundations and training that parents give their children is taking into account values, thoughts, behavior, and impact positively on children, educating with love and limits.The importance of having a good parenting style is to be clear about the objectives of education to implement, we have different relationships between parents, caregivers and guardians, as well as different ideas about education and many of them are influenced by attachment styles or raise well established emotional bonds. As parents one has the main task of helping in the development of the child; we must keep in mind that all our actions will affect in some way their ability to socialize in the future; therefore, the parenting style used will influence in a negative or positive way, being that it is how parents raise their children, in addition to giving enough tools for their development. According to Mantilla (2019):"Broadly speaking, this parenting approach focuses on respect for children's physiological and maturational processes and consideration of their secure attachment needs provided by a family environment suited to these ends." (p.62). The physical, biological and physiological features that are taken into account for the infant's development will have an important starting point based on understanding and respecting the path it takes, the time required for each process and the child's knowledge and learning to carry out developmental activities to achieve the potential of his or her abilities.The positive parenting style is another way of educating from home and within the classroom, being implemented recently, these terms of parenting styles had not had great impact until UNICEF recognized the rights of children, thus worrying about the environment in which children grow and develop, ie the type of education they were given, and how parents and guardians, correct or considered as a form of punishment, now it is considered better to give them a dignified treatment to children and to give them the right to be treated with dignity and dignity.In this way they will develop for themselves the ability to understand and separate good from bad actions and their consequences.Then, the positive or respectful parenting style will result in the interaction of the child with its environment, how it develops naturally and will not be guided based on the decisions of the adult, since this would result in the same way of traditional parenting, The important thing to emphasize in this type of parenting is that it is no longer based on blows or belittling, but the main point is love and respect to educate children without leaving aside the limits, with this the children understand when the actions are wrong and assume the consequences, but are not violated for having done them.Positive parenting takes into consideration that, if the child receives respect, love, is considered a participant in family decisions and not as a child is usually taken, simply as a spectator, he will feel good, therefore, he will have a good behavior, since his feelings are valued, the child will take his responsibilities with encouragement; besides, these always depend on his maturity; forming the character of a responsible and reflexive adult. The management of rules (limits) and sanctions (or consequences): when there are clear, non-excessive rules in the families, discussed with or explained to the children, it is easier to recognize their compliance and manage non-compliance. It is important that, in the event of non-compliance with the rule, consequences or sanctions are proposed that are coherent with the offense, short, consistent, explained or agreed upon with the children, so that they can be used at the time and avoid that The child's behavior reaches the point where the parent "no longer knows what to do" and resorts to hitting or yelling (Isaza, 2011, p. 14).Limits have a crucial point in this parenting style, as the parent is not subject to the child and his rules, but works on the basis of limiting, being the parent firm in decisions and consequences so that the child can see a difference between him and his caregiver, therefore, if there is the required respect, then the adult must have the patience demanded not to fall into exasperation.Physical or degrading punishment will only make the child not know how to express mixed feelings by not being able to feel safe and loved, for this positive parenting seeks to replace punishments or blows with more humanistic and concrete alternatives for the development of children, in order to have responsible adults and aware of their actions, based on all the actions that are seen every day, since the child will no longer be surrounded by a hostile environment, but, on the contrary, will have the confidence to be himself and express himself without fear of being belittled.In relation to the parenting style used during toilet training, it will take into account the time the child takes to learn, emphasizing that it is not a limiting factor, but it does have a great influence; for this we can also recognize that parenting styles talk about the bond that the parent will have with their children and the attachment they should have, for this we must know what bonds and attachment are and which is beneficial for the child and which can damage or stop the development.

1.4.1 Affective links.

We refer to an affective bond, to the feeling generated between a caregiver who does not necessarily have a blood relationship with the infant, i.e., friends, acquaintances, teachers, educators, or tutors, this bond is generated through trust between the infant and the adult, although it is mentioned that the bond can be generated by adults, or people of the same age, which is generated by the trust and security that can be projected to the infant.That is, the 3 year old child is discovering the world at this time of knowledge and self-discovery, he feels that many things generate fear or anxiety, that is why having a person to support him, motivate him, take care of him, makes him feel comfortable and protected, this will help him to trust in what he does and the decisions he makes, because he will be in a loving environment.The importance of teaching a bond to the child is to be part of their growth and show them empathy, care for themselves and the care they should have for others, the child to learn this will also generate it in their family circle or school context to require this type of bond will be necessary in their daily lives so that the people responsible for their care should generate this requirement.The link is mainly linked to the autonomy that we want to generate in the child, since if at home the child is given the security and confidence he/she needs for new experiences, he/she will not be afraid or anxious when trying out new activities and activities that are new to him/her. On the contrary, he will have the desire to support those around him, because he will create in him the ability to be empathetic; the link will have to do when the child is in an environment of communication, since in order to create the link he will have to establish a relationship with the person, generating that trust with the person who has affinity with him.The bond, unlike attachment, is that the bond can occur with any external person who does not have a blood tie, and attachment is always generated with one of the infant's biological parents, it can be described as the bond shared as a result of the biological formation that the child has. Attachments can occur mostly with the mother, since she is the caregiver and carrier of the fetus, at the beginning of the human life process, this attachment is generated in a physical way with the umbilical cord, after that an emotional bond of the mother with the baby develops. As such, the bond encompasses the relationship that the child will have with his or her caregivers and will depend on how he or she treats, involves, supports, helps, so that the child can generate trust and security in him or her; but this will not be gained overnight, but there must be a relationship and a coexistence so that the child can originate the bond.

1.4.2 Attachment

Having said this, then we will recognize attachment, how it is, and what benefits it has, we will begin by saying that there are several types of attachment in which many times we could already talk about something unhealthy or attention to exceed The normal for attachment; therefore, it is important to know some of them, which we will know in detail later on. Specifically, attachment is the human being's way of developing a close or intimate relationship with a person other than himself, in which it is said that the relationship will be lasting, stable and trusting, usually it takes a long time to achieve that attachment, so that as human beings we can strengthen ourselves emotionally, attachment is a relevant point because it will determine how we relate in society with others and will give us the necessary confidence and autonomy; emphasizing that it must be a healthy attachment so that it can give positive results.According to Bowlby (1980), attachment is what the child needs to have a positive emotional development in which all his or her needs are met, and he emphasizes that a close relationship with parents who meet these needs will result in good mental health in children.Based on studies by child psychoanalyst John Bowlby, it was reported that "in (1980) he studied 44 children institutionalized for theft. In all cases there was evidence of previous experiences of abuse and maltreatment by parents." (Moneta, 2014, p. 265).Mental health outcomes were deplorable, as they had no parents to meet their needs while suffering physical abuse.The attachment theory in a current approach allows us to ensure that a secure attachment, with a stable and continuous caregiver, can ensure an adequate cognitive and mental development of the child who will become an adult, even taking into account genetic risks. Moreover, primary attachments become of primary importance in old age and also in conditions of physical or mental impairment or disability at any age (Moneta, 2014, p.p. 265, 266).Any attitude or effect of the way of being will also be the result of the attachment that the child had mainly from the parents, if it was a healthy attachment or had some negative effect, therefore, let us emphasize that attachment should not only be given in early childhood, but must be strengthened over time because attachment is necessary at all difficult times and it is good to know that you can count on someone to support you emotionally.

1.4.2 Types of attachment

Secure attachment refers to the fact that both the child and the parent seek protection and security by requiring that all needs be met. Children who develop this type of attachment will be emotionally stable in the future, relate more easily and tend to have better developed relationships.The avoidant attachment type consists of the parent or caregiver not attending to the child's needs, so the child will grow up in a fragile environment, emotionally, in need of attention and as an adult will have problems in The child will therefore be affected if he/she is treated with this type of attachment.Another type of attachment is the ambivalent attachment, which is characteristic due to the fact that people who suffer it tend to react with anguish, fear, anger to separation, since emotionally they will have deficiencies because they did not have the teaching of such values in childhood, besides the fact that they always lacked someone to cover their needs.Disorganized attachment is that the caregiver has attitudes that confuse the child, since the behavior will be unpredictable for the child and will create confusion in their emotions and way of acting, they are usually children who have problems relating to others and tend to destroy toys and be aggressive, because at home is what they have learned only physical, emotional damage because they are constantly spoken to with insults resulting in emotional inconsistency.The attachment of parents is the bond of consanguineous with the paternal figure, in this process of sphincter control support, the confidence generated by the paternal attachment in children is a great support, more than for a gender characteristic, it is for a physiological characteristic, that is to say, both recognize that they have a penis, this is how in this type of attachment we can generate greater confidence to be able to teach a child to go to the bathroom. We must take into account that attachment and bonds are different, so we will know why they are different, but they are related and are of utmost importance for children, according to Burutxaga et al. (2018) can take of importance and natural type of attachment: This purely biological conceptualization of attachment gave way to a more comprehensive interpretation in which Bowlby spoke not only of physical proximity, but also of "permanent availability" of the main figure (Bowlby, 1988). This availability is not exclusively of a physical nature (being located in space close to the child) but also poses a need for an adequate emotional response on the part of this main figure. The child's internalization of the main figure as available and capable of responding emotionally is the key to the development of a secure attachment system (pp. 1- 2).

1.4.3 Differences between bonding and attachment.

As we could see, the characteristics of attachment and bonding are very similar, but they are not the same, since one refers more to a natural need of the child with parental figures and the other is related to the people surrounding the child; positive attachment these days is gaining momentum thanks to the response it has in children in their behavior and how they relate to others when they are treated with love and respect, so it can be helpful for the adult, having strategies to develop attachment, to cover primordial needs such as the relationship between child and parents. The bond, on the other hand, is directed to the emotional development, the human being knows how to relate naturally, therefore, the bond requires more relationship with the mother, mainly because behaviors in newborn children The mother is the one who has to make up for these basic needs and begins to have a closer relationship with her child, this relationship is considered attachment and will have consequences in the adult life of this person and how he/she creates a relationship with those around him/her; the bond needs to be developed in a good way because it is developed in early childhood and has repercussions in the future.Although attachment and bonding are closely related, they are not the same, since bonding makes the child know what it is to relate to others other than himself or the parents, having a relationship that indicates some place, some conversation, will make the person be linked to another by having this in common; it establishes limits since it could be taken as belonging to be linked, but emphasizes that in some relationships can be terminated, therefore, the bond would end in most but not all, for example "divorced parents have children in common as a link".Attachment develops in the first months of life and is mainly developed by the parents, since it corresponds to how the first relationship with the parents was established and how the child will grow, with what idea he/she will develop and also what type of attachment the child will have and how this will affect his/her future and the bonds the child will develop with the people around him/her and the importance he/she will give to these bonds.

This attachment relationship is always established between the child and another person; it is not possible to include a third person in this duality. Although it is possible for the child to develop two distinct and qualitatively different attachment relationships, it is not possible to include a third party in this duality. The idea of a group attachment is underdeveloped, but it is not well developed. The idea of group attachment is underdeveloped.The bond, on the other hand, does not seem to be limited to a dual relationship or to a specific number of people with whom it can be formed; it is open to be formed between several people. The bond can be established with several people at the same time or even with a group of people, regardless of the number of members with whom a space, a goal or a hope is shared, and in which the bond acts as a link between all of them (Burutxaga et al., 2018, p.12).Therefore, attachment will serve to learn to relate to others, starting with the relationship with parents, beginning to generate bonds with those around the individual, whether many or few people, and the emotional development that these bonds will help the child.This chapter made us go inside and recognize that development has a time and a natural maturation, therefore, we must recognize and let nature act, recognize what we are talking about when addressing the issue of toilet training and the time it takes to start the process; how the relationship with parents called attachment will have an impact on the development of the child, touching on such issues makes us have enough time to learn how to control the child's bowel and bladder; how the relationship with parents called attachment will have an impact on the development of the child, touching on such issues makes us have enough time to learn how to control the child's bowel and bladder. knowledge to take to the next level the support to be given to the child and to recognize the time needed and how to generate a support network for the child.

CHAPTER 2

LET'S TALK ABOUT SPHINCTER CONTROL.

We discovered that education is not something that the teacher does, but that it is a natural process that develops spontaneously in the human being.
- Maria Montessori

Toilet training is a natural process that can be simple and uncomplicated if the child has a mature brain, physical and nervous system. We can recognize that in a newborn there is a voiding reflex that is not controlled by the child and as the child grows this reflex will be controlled. The level of language is also a factor that influences the process of bowel and bladder control, since in this way children will express what they need; finally, psychological maturity will allow the child to recognize the signals that his body gives them to evacuate at necessary times and in private, therefore, we must be patient to provide the necessary experiences for them to experience and recognize when the child is obtaining the necessary maturity. Children can stop diapering according to the degree of stimulation and when they are biologically, psychologically and affectively mature to do so. Parents should be aware that the neuromuscular function that leads to bladder control takes a period between 2 to 3 years of age as a reference, although few children achieve bladder control. complete before the age of 3. Since each child and his circumstances are particular and unfolds within a sociocultural environment that determines it (Cárdenas, 2016, p.10).As we can see, the sociocultural environment also has a guideline in the sphincter control, because this will often determine the relationship between parents or more closely with the mother, this is because society considers that the mother is the pillar for the accompaniment of the child, because she is the one who, in theory, generates more confidence in the infant, is more patient, knows her child better, has better tactics, reality is that the father is also an important part of the accompaniment, because the child gets the motivation to start this process when he sees that both parents are involved and have the interest that the child can learn it; Remembering that it is the parents' job to accompany the child, therefore, the parents can be asked to teach the child through imitation; for example, if the learner is a boy, the father can be asked to show him how he should do it by taking him to the bathroom, showing him how he does it, as opposed to the girl who will imitate her mother by sitting down. The child will always be able to learn from the example given by his parents, of course we will base ourselves on the fact that every process gives guidelines to recognize if it is possible to start, therefore, we will know how to start with the training, giving the support that the child needs.

2.1 When sphincter control begins.

When we talk about sphincter control, we talk about patience, love, routine, certain values that must also be instilled and set an example, for example, by Of course, 100% mastered control will take time and will require support; understanding that traditional teachings or behavioral teaching speaking more specifically, generate learning, but this is more squared because it is something based on reward and punishment, so in the accompaniment of toilet training we speak more of a mature learning and autonomy, pointing Garcia (2017), "To encourage this, and thanks to science, we know that children are very predisposed to memorize what interests them, being active and engaged, making mistakes and repeating themselves as many times as they need to, despite the passion and extraordinary commitment of our teachers, this maladaptive system interferes with the development of individual potentials, "with the human potentials that we all have at birth - oral, social, linguistic, mathematical, emotional, cognitive, creative" (p.1), therefore, this type of teaching could affect the process, therefore, toilet training should be adapted in a novel and easy way for children.From Skinner's perspective, traditional teaching has certain deficiencies that hinder learning. One of them is that it provides the student with more aversive consequences than positive ones. Other frequent flaws are the sequencing of instructional materials and collective instruction. The recognition of these flaws led Skinnner to raise a series of considerations accepted during the 1960s and 1970s, under the heading of programmed teaching (González, 2004, p. 15). There is a great majority of people who grew up with behaviorist teaching, which resulted in learning, but most of the time in an unpleasant way or with negative stimuli for the learners, taking into account that all children have different types of learning, the teaching should be adapted for everyone so that it can be beneficial and simple.According to the stages of development by Erick Erikson (1963), sphincter control will depend on the conditions in which the child has developed, if he has grown with autonomy and dependence on his parents or if he has grown with doubt and shame, the way in which he learns to control his sphincters will depend on this: if he was pressured with blows, insults or humiliations or if the correct time of the body and maturation was respected to achieve a natural advance and in his own time.Montessori (as cited in Cárdenas, 2016) Children learn on their own and our role as parents is to respect them as the individuals they are and provide them with a prepared environment in which to develop their potential. If we extrapolate the principles of the method to sphincter control, we will need to facilitate access to the bathroom and respect their dignity and time. In other words, the child is not trained to give up the diaper, using behaviorist methods based on rewards and punishments so that the child ceases a certain behavior (using a diaper), but rather we try to provide the appropriate environment for the child to become aware of how to control his body functions (Muñoz, 2022, p. 1). So parents do not make the child learn, but the task of the parents is to create an environment conducive to the proper development of sphincter control, also emphasizing that a simple help could make deplorable the progress that has already been obtained, because the child will not feel sufficient to achieve this process and will necessarily need the support of their parents becoming dependent on them.The importance of the process is to know how the development of the body works physically and neurologically, the physiological needs that the child must develop in order to start the process using medical terms could be taken as the need for maturity and to know how these changes are and how we can recognize when they happen.[2]

It is considered important to start sphincter control at 2 years of age, tentatively, as long as the child reaches maturity, and respecting the individual characteristics of each child, i.e., if the child needs to stop diapering, we first take into account what he can already achieve such as: control over his legs, being able to pass liquid from one container to another by himself, not wetting his diaper for a long period of time, feeling discomfort with the diaper on or when he defecates, etc. The following factors should also be taken into account:Speech stimulation: if the child expresses orally or manages to express the need to go to the bathroom, the child will begin to give signs to announce that he/she is already dirty, short words such as: poop or pee-pee, and many times the child will start to say it. will scream, maybe parents will be uncomfortable at the beginning, but we must understand that this is a totally normal aspect.Personal autonomy: The child's ability to think as an individual being, to take actions on his own, that is, he is already aware of his decision, therefore, the child will be able to pull down his underwear and pull it up, to try to get dressed, to go to the right place to relieve himself, to be able to perform tasks typical of children of his age; at the beginning we must support him all the time to pull down his clothes so he can relieve himself and emphasize that he can do it, so that little by little he does not need more help and he himself is aware of what he is capable of. Initial motivation: It is an aspect where the child will be interested in what is coming in the future, the child's interest will determine that their learning will be more concise; the child's interest in using the bathroom or the curiosity to accompany the parents to the bathroom to begin to recognize the elements that surround the toilet, such as toilet paper, sink, etc. is born. By doing this, the child will be encouraged to enter and will gradually lose his or her fear; in addition, parents should provide the necessary support when setting up the bathroom to improve the child's experience.We must learn to recognize the signs when a child is ready, physically, emotionally and psychologically, to begin the process of toilet training. Of course, when children do not learn or have difficulty learning, parents do not think that they have not yet matured well, but rather feel guilty for not meeting expectations or that they are not raising them well.For this reason we are emphasizing the support offered to parents first so that they know when to start, that they should notice in their children and recognize that it is not an overnight process and that it requires a lot of patience, in addition to the social pressure or competition that children often experience between families is indicative of abuse to do well because the consequence will be that they will not do well and only damage their integrity.The age of onset of bladder (urinary) and anal sphincter control varies from one child to another, but in general terms ranges from 18 to 24 months, in fact, this depends on the degree of maturity and development of muscles and nerves that make possible the voluntary control of the sphincters; defecation control usually comes before bladder sphincter control, which may start as discomfort of the child in the presence of a dirty diaper, this is more marked when there is fecal matter, tolerating a wet diaper with urine for a longer time. (Cerón, 2010 p.1).The age is not a determinant, since it will always depend on what the child requires, if it can be recognized that the child has sufficient skills to leave the diaper can begin with the process of accompaniment, but it should be borne in mind that absolutely always the child is the one who gives signs that already can stop diapering, considering their maturity and the developmental milestones they have already reached.How can we recognize that the child is ready to begin the process of sphincter control in a natural way, the child will give indications that the diaper makes him/her uncomfortable, the learning of defecation occurs first and it will always depend on the stimulus given, the environment provided and the pressure, emphasizing that the age at which they begin always varies, taking as a reference that the process begins from 18 to 24 months, but it is not something established by force because it will depend on the maturation.

Parents must look at their child and recognize the peculiarities he/she enjoys, respecting his/her rhythms, needs and potentialities. And the child, in addition to having the physiological conditions, must meet others: a cognitive development that allows establishing a verbal communication channel (understanding and using words linked to need), that is able to imitate, to realize his sensations, to feel interested in learning proposals, to establish connections (dry/pleasant) (Moya, 2013, p.1). (Moya, 2013, p.1). It is important that all those involved with the child are supportive of the parents, as it will be in the hands of everyone to support the child to achieve the objective, looking for strategies such as giving the child the confidence to warn and that he/she can be taken to the toilet. The child's caregivers, whether family members or educators, should then be asked to provide support to create a good environment for the children so that the child will have a support network to feel confident about the process that is about to begin without threats or pressure.A crucial aspect to emphasize is that you should not start the process if the child is going through a considerable change such as the arrival of a sibling, a divorce, an illness, as this affects him emotionally, why he feels displaced, forgotten, makes him experience a lot of sadness, in addition to the feeling of loss and emptiness, therefore, it will affect the physical environment, It is important to emphasize that we should not limit the child in the process, but rather understand that it will help him to be autonomous, to feel good because he will make the first decisions of his life, so as caregivers we only have to accompany him, but not make decisions about him.The society in which we live is complicated. The incorporation of women into the world of work has set in motion the phenomenon of kindergartens and schooling at very early ages (3 years), in classes that work with many children. In these circumstances, it is very difficult to respect the individual needs of each child: for educational institutions, it is more practical to treat them all the same, to standardize the daily routines and processes of the children as much as possible.Everyone has to eat at the same time, pee in the toilet and sleep at the same time. siesta at their own time and without help. In other words, the system needs very autonomous children, because it cannot find any other way to take care of them while mom and dad work (Ros, 2022, p.1).In society, children are constantly under incredible pressure, whether it is for walking, what kind of milk they drink, how long it took them to talk, who gets better grades, who is more

skilled, how long it took them to leave the diaper, without realizing it, we exert a pressure that they should not experience, We are so much affected that instead of supporting them and trusting in the process and maturation of children, we make them accelerate their growth and have attitudes and experiences that do not go according to their age, of course this leads to problems from a very young age that, although we do not believe it, are the result of wanting to fit into society.The process of sphincter control has several points to consider to start it as the balance that can be taken as body control to perform certain activities such as running without falling, hold an object and walk without throwing the object and for example, if the child already manages to jump with both feet, Similarly, it would be an indication to leave the diaper, discomfort, the fact that the child begins to tell if he/she has already gone to the bathroom, if he/she already recognizes where to relieve him/herself, if he/she hides to relieve him/herself or asks for privacy, would be some crucial points to recognize that it is time to start with the process.Encouraging children in many ways, for example, by celebrating the accomplishment of a waste in the potty or toilet bowl generates confusion in the little ones is to feel proud and want to show it to everyone, without a sense of shame or embarrassment for what has been done, which often crosses the limits of decency, ie try to show it at any time, sometimes this also generates a repression of this because it is uncomfortable for them to present to others or perform the same activity, This process will often depend on the maturation of physiological, biological, and psychological form, as a recommendation for parents, is to encourage the process without falling into the prize of the exhibition and give guidance on the places that is correct to perform this activity.
same needs.

2.2 Consequences of poor accompaniment

As parents or teachers, many times we make mistakes when starting the process of toilet training due to lack of knowledge, social pressure, or work indications, therefore, we do not realize the damage that we can generate, as it can be brutal, because it will not only affect the emotional area, behavioral area, but also in health and for that it is important to know what are the actions, a bad accompaniment.At the beginning of the control, the child is limited to ingesting food or drinks until a certain time, because many times parents seek information that they can take from any unreliable internet page, but ingesting drinks will make the child experience sensations such as having a full bladder, feel like peeing or pooping, so following advice from any page makes the methods doubtful and in these times it is easier to find information that was not available at the beginning of the control process. manipulated by anyone, then it will affect the child unknowingly, as the parents will believe that they are supporting the child.This topic mainly talks about the ignorance that surrounds sphincter control, since it has brought irreparable difficulties and incredible setbacks over the years, such as urine problems in adolescents and behavioral setbacks such as wanting to put on diapers again; sphincter control was taken so lightly that it did not matter if the child learned it well or not, since it was only something that had to be learned without caring about what methods to use and whether they would harm the child, besides not seeking the child's welfare, but simply that he/she would do it.Something shocking is that due to the lack of knowledge on the subject, many parents resorted or still do to cruel and insensitive methods such as beatings, intimidation, humiliation, for example: they could leave the child with wet clothes as a method of punishment and thus understand that it was not right what he was doing, make him pick up or even wash his dirty clothes so that he would have a retaliation, this had as a consequence important emotional and social problems; comparisons between relatives or acquaintances, thinking that this will make the child get tired and once and for all learn, however, it is making the child feel contempt and show less interest or no interest at all to leave the diaper. (Bezos & Escribano, 2012).When we force the situation, we are forced to sit the child on the potty every moment or remind them every so often that they have to go to the bathroom. If the child needs this dependence on the adult to avoid wearing a diaper, is that it is not yet ready. It can become counterproductive, since we generate an overprotection that can degenerate into a need for dependence to go to the bathroom and self-control is neglected (Palacios, 2019, p.1).

The result of a bad accompaniment can affect adults to such a level that they can have traumas, due to the fact that they had a bad experience and even experience fear when they have accidents on their clothes; A 10 year old child who has problems to hold his urine or at night he goes to the bathroom in bed and gives indications that he cannot move or does not wake up, may show us that the problem behind this is that he had a bad accompaniment of sphincter control and may have experienced violence during the process and therefore experiences fear, because when he was discovered the accompanying adults had outbursts of anger when they saw that he soiled himself and hit or humiliated the child.It is of utmost importance to emphasize that the beginning of the accompaniment must be in an enriching environment for the child, a friendly environment, with empathy and make the child see that we do not want him to learn as we were taught to many adults, in a hostile environment, with beatings, humiliations and comparisons, because that is how society wanted it, on the contrary, he must be careful of these attitudes and behaviors or beatings because this is totally reprehensible; because this learning is something he must do throughout his life and until his last days, therefore, let us help him to learn freely and happily.There are also rumors in society that the best time to initiate the process and to accompany the sphincter control should be done in summer when it is hot, for the comfort of the parents, because the child will have more ease to perform his needs, he will not be cold, it will not hurt him, etc. when this can be taken merely as something superficial rather the easiest thing is sought, since in summer there is less skin irritation, more heat to dry the clothes, etc.There are some health issues to consider. Excessively wet skin and contact with urine and feces can cause diaper rash. Because cloth diapers cannot prevent moisture on your baby's skin as well as disposable diapers, it is especially important to change cloth diapers promptly after your baby wets or soils. (American Academy of Pediatrics, 2013, p.1).Taking into account the stimulus that the child receives from a cloth diaper or a disposable diaper is different because with the cloth diaper, as it is not absorbent or does not have chemicals that the child feels comfortable with, it will increase the discomfort and seek to change the diaper or leave it for good, which could be taken as positive for the cloth diaper and can be taken as beneficial for the child.Remembering that this is a maturing process, it will be taken into account if the child has the need or we see characteristics such as discomfort with the diaper, begins to warn and even if the diaper is removed on its own, we are in the station. our duty is to accompany and support the child, so that we remove ourselves from the thoughts of society and let the natural flow.We come to find defiant children or temperaments difficult to control that many times the failure to establish limits and rules at home harm the indications of the authorities, that is to say to command or suggest where they can and can not do the needs, as often children as a form of challenge to authority do not want to warn and is done by the corridors of the house or in the clothes, currently has a great protection to the rights, and it is not easy to set a limit, since at the time the corrections to these acts could be with a spanking.Seeing the other side of the coin we can understand that noble children can be treated, but if a bad accompaniment is done, it can be harmful at an emotional and social level, since it will damage their self-esteem and autonomy, since they will be afraid to ask permission to go to the toilet or even to participate in activities, on the other hand, if we face a child with a difficult temperament they will have some difficulty in setting limits, so parents should be careful about how to carry out the accompaniment of toilet training.

However, since children have many rights and associations that protect them, it is emphasized that it is necessary to know that as parents it is no longer as before that you could beat them, humiliate them without any problem, since this was the way to educate, now children have besides parents, someone else to take care of them and protect them. This is also talked about in the classrooms, a child can express himself freely in a classroom, with the nanny, with the other relatives, etc. and thus expose the problems he/she is living at home; as we could see nowadays, many of the children are taken to daycare centers because both parents work, then the children have more people to love and protect them, so the parents are exposed to be arrested, judged, etcetera for doing these actions if a child is affected by society simply for not learning sphincter control fast, the parents will be much more judged and exposed to hit the child or do any action that threatens his/her integrity. It is important to help get rid of the taboos that revolve around this process, because of course everything has consequences and not only affect the children, but also the parents, siblings, and family surrounding the child, it is important to recognize that giving the child enough tools and confidence in him and his maturation processes will make him seek autonomy to do it alone and thus succeed.In the following, we will learn about some problems that are the result of a bad accompaniment, at what level they can affect the child and if they can be solved or treated.

2.2.1 Encopresis

Encopresis is referred to as a sphincter control disorder in which the child does not control the elimination of stool, which begins by the Constipation is very common in children and in clinics, because when the child begins to control sphincter the child may have problems to assimilate what is the process and his body and unconscious not wanting to get dirty or have the discomfort of having accidents tends to hold the urge and not go to the bathroom, this will result in constipation, which in the beginning is normal, but much depends on the parents to be aware that can skip the step of constipation and does not become something more serious or chronic that later will have to be followed up by a doctor.Supporting the child so that he/she can lose fear and have the freedom to relieve him/herself at his/her own time is relevant so that control can be achieved, thus taking care of his/her emotional health and having tools to obtain better results and firm bases from which he/she will not have setbacks or repercussions to health, such as encopresis.According to the National Library of Medicine (2022) "If a child over the age of 4 has been toilet trained, but still defecates and soils his or her clothes, this is called encopresis. The child may or may not be doing this on purpose" (p.1). Encopresis is when an older child does not control his or her stool normally and without withholding soiling, i.e., he or she has not mastered 100 percent control.Encopresis tends to be embarrassing for the child who suffers from it, which causes him to hide the leaks he has had by performing actions such as smearing it anywhere, hiding his dirty underwear, etc. This disorder occurs because medically speaking according to Stanford Children's Hospital (2022) "Stool accumulates (impacted) in the rectum and large intestine (colon). Stool cannot move forward. The rectum and bowel become enlarged due to hard, impacted stool. Over time, liquid stool may begin to leak around the hard, dry, impacted stool." (p.1) this will cause children to suffer from rejection, punishment, humiliation, which most of the time worsen the situations.The good news is that the treatment emphasizes the accompaniment of the parents, a relevant point is that the better the accompaniment, the faster the reduction of this disorder will be achieved, relatively the treatment is more experimental, since the results that have been obtained have been from real situations with patients suffering from this disorder, The importance of knowing that this disorder is often not the result of the pressure exerted on the child, or the parents if they are carrying a good accompaniment, but is the result of the change accepted by the child, pain when defecating as a result of a junk diet and their way of retaining stool, encopresis can be overcome with medical treatment, therapeutic plan, an accompaniment and guidance to sphincter control, and so on. So encopresis if it has a solution always based on what caused it and how willing we are to support the child to overcome this wrong step, taking into account that it is also a result of the child's diet and the fear of defecating because of the pain caused by the stool, taking into account that the child's socioeconomic status will have a great impact on the child's health. influence, but this does not mean that it will be determinant for your health, trust will play an important role in this problem. In some cases there are children who due to distrust of the teacher do not ask or tell her that they want to go to the toilet or do not feel comfortable at school because they prefer the privacy of their home, then they tend to put up with it and as a result there is encopresis to which parents blame mostly to school or teachers when they have not worked confidence at home to perform their needs at school which is already like their second home and prevent these health problems. Next, we will learn about a disorder aimed at potty training.

2.2.1 Enuresis.

This disorder is directed to urinary elimination, since there is no control of this, so there are accidents or inability to control urine, either during the day, at naptime or night, which we can say that at first is normal for this should have a complete analysis and with great care of the child this is the task of parents and caregivers to recognize if it is evolving well control or should have a visit to the pediatrician.

According to Irurtia (2022):

"The chronological age from which it is considered a problem is five years, in the case of girls, and six years in the case of boys, or an equivalent level of development. These are approximate ages, since it is considered that the organic maturity for sphincter control is around three years of age". (P.7). According to this, total control of urination in a child is tentatively given until the age of six years, therefore, the child has not yet reached full maturity to have a mastery, also it can be expected that during the nap or night there is no control and leakage occurs.When there is no bladder control, commonly called bedwetting, there are variations of why this is happening, the sphincter control happens by muscle which needs to be exercised to master it, therefore, the child does not have sufficient maturity and training to control it, plus the bladder has a lot to do, as it must be sufficiently developed to contain urine in long periods such as bedtime.When this disorder lasts longer than expected it is important to diagnose with a specialist such as a psychiatrist, then he will give a correct treatment for this problem, we can combine emotional problems as a trigger for this problem, since it is used as a quick way out or to get attention, It is interesting to note that even the lifestyle affects the child because as seen above children are exposed to high levels of excessive pressure and result in problems such as bedwetting, an example of this is a 5 year old boy who does not want to warn for shame does not go to the toilet.This, coupled with not drinking enough water, results in a child with a urinary tract infection who has intense pain when urinating and emotional distress. Treatment for this health problem is merely accompanying and in more extreme cases medical treatment, according to Ortíz (2018): "The bladder expansion method of Kimmel and Kimmel (1970): Most useful in daytime enuresis. It uses positive reinforcement of intervals and increasing amounts of retained urine in a measured bucket. The urinary alarm (pipi-stop) of Mowrer (1978): It has the highest success rate of all existing treatments (75-80%). It basically consists of a circuit that sounds a buzzer when the child begins to urinate. It is recommended to use it together with overlearning, making the Child consume 1/4 liter of water before going to bed several nights and turning on the alarm intermittently (every other day). "(p.1).

As we can see, there are effective methods that help to improve the disorder or eliminate it, so we can accompany the child to improve this problem or overcome it definitively so that the child has more confidence in him and what he can achieve.

2.2.3 Setbacks

In all the progress that the child has already had there is the possibility of a setback of what has been learned and this can happen for various situations, the child's development takes a process and a series of steps that are normal and can be checked, a useful tool to know if the child is taking a development within the normal are the developmental milestones which will give us a starting point to balance between what is normal and what we should pay special attention to. Developmental development is not a homogeneous and linear process. Regressions are normal and occur quite frequently, especially in the stage from 3 to 5 years old, in the transition to preschool. Children may be searching for lost security, may require care, protection or attention. It usually coincides with a difficult moment or a process of change in the child's life, such as the birth of a brother or sister, a change of address, starting school, separation from parents, or some loss. But also sometimes it is simply a necessary stop to continue evolving (Center for Pediatric Specialties, 2018, p.1). As we can see, it is completely normal for a child to regress, so we may have to start again with the accompaniment to make him/her feel safe; the fact that emotionally he/she is unstable will have a lot to do with it, since as we saw before, for a child who has yet to develop his/her emotions, to know how to control them, besides the fact that it is difficult for them to accept such drastic changes quickly, they seek help or attention in this way, so we must pay special attention to the setbacks so that as caregivers we can meet the needs that he/she requires. Similarly, a regression is a sign that the child has not yet developed the needs that are essential for the onset of toilet training, such as physiological, cognitive, language, emotional, social and social needs, etcetera; parents have the duty to ask themselves why this setback occurred if there was a change in the child's routine, if he/she is going through a drastic change, if it was started at an inappropriate age[3] or too hurriedly, in this way parents can recognize and support the aspect to work on and resume the training for control. When the process is already learned, put into practice and suddenly there is a setback, it is frustrating for parents, so they tend to no longer want to continue with the training, or do it, but already in an abrupt way, hurting the child's feelings, making him feel unimportant and with little capacity, therefore, instead of enjoying, continue with the training, he will feel insecure to warn and fall into a vicious circle where even parents can become violent, because they will have problems of anger and frustration to stay stagnant.The poop control process takes longer and can last up to six years. For this reason, you should always keep a close eye on your little one and not get angry with him if he regresses in toilet training. In most cases, these setbacks are usually due to a change in one of the following areas: "Personal": toilet training makes children feel older; therefore, they may be afraid and feel unprepared.

"Family": a divorce, the arrival of a sibling or a death are causes that alter your routine."School": the first days of school or the change of a teacher can provoke a certain state of nerves in your child. Although at the beginning it may be an event that awakens a lot of excitement in the child, with the passage of time it can lead to concern."Social": problems related to their friends or peers can influence them in the same way as comparisons (Lopez, 2021, p.1).As we can see, regressions are to some extent normal, but it is up to the parents to examine the child's situation and what could have happened or is happening to cause this regression, ask for professional help, it never hurts to take the child to the pediatrician to verify that there is no other problem that is affecting the child, as it may also involve physical causes associated with diseases or infections, therefore, it may require treatment. A crucial point is to be attentive to what caused the setback, not only the parents can be taken as supporters, but also the people around the child such as teachers, grandparents, aunts, etc., because sometimes parents have no interest in this issue, so it is important that as a support network the child can feel safe with people who know they are supporting him and feel capable of what he can do and take up again. Next, we will learn about how toilet training is taken in some disorders and how, although it takes a little more time, it can be achieved.

2.2.4 Sphincter control in disorders.

Toilet training is also extremely relevant in children with learning disabilities, knowing how the process is when children have psychological disorders helps us to understand how toilet training is developed in them, learning disabilities tend to delay the process because as they usually have neurological problems it may take longer to fully master it, it can be achieved one hundred percent with much support from parents and patience as we already know is a process that requires maturation of the body to develop it.Underlining that the sphincter control depends on the maturation of the nervous system and with it several factors such as physiological, language, etc. a comparison could be made with the development that the child undergoes from birth and in the course of the months, to hold the head, roll, sit, etc.; we could think that it is the same way that the training will be carried with children who have intellectual disabilities, the reality is that this will have to depend on parents, professionals, their support network, which will have to support it.Children who have a learning barrier have a different or slower process in developing certain skills, therefore, we must not wait for the child to show signs, because we could not know if it is ready or not, then you should start to push the child to start learning to go to the bathroom at an age that motivates the rest of the children, we are talking about approximately 2 years and older, this to stimulate and let them experience the process, It is important to emphasize that parents must know the steps to follow, because too much pressure on the child or not giving importance to the training could lead to later sphincter control disorders.

For Vygotsky (1978) learning stimulates development, that is, interrelations with others activate a group of internal processes that are internalized in the course of development. According to him, experience has shown that the child with a wider zone in his or her proximal development will have a better performance, and, therefore, this provides us with a more useful key than mental age to discover the dynamics of intellectual progress (Robles, 2018, p.81).

According to the author Vygotsky, learning with others can be a stimulus, since it also encourages the child to want to do the activities, to lose fear or insecurity, because being accompanied will be easier, if the child first experiences what will happen and not just start without prior knowledge, he/she can have a more concrete and successful learning. So starting this training in a group or with the same treatment is beneficial, making both parents and children aware of what is going to happen or how the process will be carried out can be much easier, since they will know the terrain, so to speak; now let's emphasize that the stimulus has an important role in this issue, since it will be the means by which learning will take place.Considering the support of a pediatrician or an assistance center for children with intellectual disabilities should be a must, as this will be a starting point for both parents and children, as this is where the support for the child and guidance for the parents begins and they know exactly what they should do being supported by a professional and not just by what they might see or hear anywhere.Girls and boys with intellectual disabilities, may present a series of characteristics that make the learning process slower, such as alteration in communication, difficulty to imitate, mental inflexibility; but when there are no associated physical problems or severe intellectual disability, like other girls or boys, when they acquire this learning they maintain it throughout their lives (Robles, 2018, p.1).It is a fact that starting toilet training in a child with intellectual disabilities will be a longer process, since there are characteristics that cost him/her to develop a little more, but this is not impossible, you must give the support he/she needs and a little more so that he/she can develop the necessary characteristics and can maintain this control, it should always be considered of utmost importance to go to a specialist to perform some kind of test or test that is indicative to start with the toilet training.As in all toilet training is of utmost importance to emphasize that you should not fall into attitudes that delay this learning, because as they carry a slower process, often parents fall into thinking or labeling the child as a baby or have attitudes of violence, punishment and cause fear in the child that having learning problems can have an even more serious result, For example, it will become easy or normal for him to hit his classmates, teachers, family, because it is something that he lives in his daily life and no longer takes a harmful relevance for him, but on the contrary it will be a normal issue in his life.Autonomy takes a relevant role in the life of all children, the important point here is that it goes hand in hand with sphincter control, since the result of this is that it begins to be autonomous, therefore it takes its Although it may sound like a very complicated subject because of the learning difficulties, we must understand that it is a very important subject, because when it is achieved, it gives enormous satisfaction to see and recognize the capacity of the children.

In toilet training with children who have intellectual disabilities there are methods that support parents, teachers, family, etc., such as the potty watch method which promises to be a simple method that is highly effective, because it is practically the same steps as a common training, but this should take more patience, commitment and good humor to perform all the activities that asks for at least five days to verify the child to keep notes if you have characteristics to start training and so on. One of the most successful in the United States and developed by experts is the so-called Potty Watch.This clock is programmed with a certain music or sound, depending on the child's taste. They are also adapted times when the clock sounds in a certain way. They have several types of sounds, going to the bathroom to pee, going to the bathroom to make a belly, and the time you are - in case of the second option - sitting on the toilet.

According to the experts at healthy Children.com, a website for pediatricians, children who are likely to suffer with potty training may face physical challenges,cerebral palsy, visual impairment, hearing impairment, incontinence problems, spina bifida, behavioral disorders, intellectual disabilities and developmental disorders. Depending on the child's problem, there are already several strategies that help each child to overcome this problem (QUERER Foundation, 2017, P.1).This method is specialized and used by pediatricians to give rise to the beginning of control in children with disabilities, can be adapted to the type of need of the child to let both the child and parents know the ability to advance in their development, we can even find in toy stores watches specially designed to support the training of sphincter control.

According to experts at healthyChildren.com (2015):

"Children with intellectual disabilities or developmental delays are best toilet trained one step at a time. Don't expect your child to learn to point or announce her urge to go, drop her pants, use the toilet for training, wipe herself and wash her hands all at once, just as her peers would. Toilet training will work best if you focus on the actual act of elimination first and deal with the other skills later. It is more important to keep him motivated than to achieve instant success." (p.1).This indicates that the characteristics are very similar to those of children with normal capabilities to start the process, it will undoubtedly take more time, but the crucial thing is that it will generate great satisfaction to achieve control, being always paramount good humor and patience in parents as companions to avoid frustration and carry this training in a healthy and cordial way, taking care of the integrity of the infant.We can conclude this chapter by emphasizing the pillar formed by parents, teachers, family, etc., is of utmost importance to carry a good accompaniment of toilet training, to know what not to do in the accompaniment and what consequences have bad attitudes, it is essential to recognize what characteristics to notice in children to start training, The consequences that will have repercussions on the child's health and emotionally, to finish with a very special topic that emphasizes that all children can achieve one hundred percent sphincter control, although some take a little more time, it will always generate satisfaction to see them achieve it.

CHAPTER 3
MATURATION PROCESS.

"What we see changes what we know. What we know changes, what we see."
-Jean Piaget

When we talk about accompanying the child in sphincter control training, the starting point is to wait for the child to comply with certain characteristics of development and maturation, not to rush, not to pressure, but to let what must happen flow at the time it happens, without haste, but without pause, knowing what the child must accomplish and not just wait for the sake of it, but rather to support him knowing what he must accomplish, how he must do it and with what we can stimulate in order to comply with all the processes he needs.When talking about child growth we can take 3 important topics to consider these topics are of importance because they are a fundamental part of the child's development and represent changes in his body; these points are pillars for the child's life and growth, these topics are development, maturation and growth, you might think that they are the same, but each one develops differently in the human being, in this chapter we will talk about the maturation that the child requires to start the process of sphincter control.Similarly, knowing the difference between development, maturation and growth is considerable because for growth they are crucial and related to each other, but they are not the same. It is common for both words, growth and development, as well as the concepts they express, to be intermingled and used together, since both refer to the same result: the maturation of the organism. In general, all growth entails changes in function (Cusminsky et al., 1994, p.5).Learning to differentiate between physical growth and development is important, for example, physical growth is quantitative, since we can observe and measure it, such as weight, height, understanding are some of these points, this gives us signs that the child has noticeable and visible changes to move to another stage, then the development is the one that can not be measured or observed with the naked eye, but if you can perceive, it is important to emphasize that these processes should not be parallel or grow at the same time.Development and maturation are differentiated by the fact that development is directed to the set of functions that occur in the human being, such as: the change of relevant areas such as physical, social, emotional, intellectual, he is no longer a person who is guided by others or always depend on his parents, but now he can be more independent; maturation, on the other hand, is directed more to what the child reaches when his physical and sexual development is completed and he becomes an adult. Development is evaluated in a different way, for example, with questionnaires, tests, tests, as well as a series of tests that are the developmental milestones that tell us about what the child is supposed to achieve at a certain age, how he/she achieves it, and if he/she still does not do it, what to do to support him/her. Maturation refers to what the child already knows and recognizes, what he/she is acquiring as abilities and skills and how using these will make him/her a functional adult and fully aware of what he/she does and should do, knowing that each action has a consequence for what will be his/her life later on.Speaking of maturation in a more clinical setting according to the Handbook of Child Growth and Development, Cusminsky et al. (1994):Maturation is understood as the process of progressive acquisitions of new functions and characteristics, which begins with conception and ends when the being reaches the adult state. This concept must be clearly differentiated from growth, which is characterized by an increase in size and is measured in centimeters, kilograms, etc. Maturation, on the other hand, is measured by the appearance of new functions (walking, speaking, holding the head), or events (appearance of a tooth, appearance of the first menstruation in a girl, appearance of new bones in X-rays, etc.) (p.25). (p.25).Therefore, knowing the term of clinical maturation makes us aware of what it entails; maturation is the characteristic of the human being that indicates the achievements that he has as time goes by, with each day the child acquires functions with his day to day, with the experience that he acquires from his environment, this makes his growth healthy and also gives indications if he has The difference with growth is that maturation is distinguished by acquisitions during its development.A relevant point is that each child grows differently, some have characteristics that distinguish them from others, but the maturation occurs in all equally, since when it is perceived that reached its maturity, is when it already obtained all the capabilities that form an adult, in all can occur at different times in some before, in others, but always reach it.Likewise, maturation is divided in different ways such as dental maturation when they begin to change milk teeth for permanent teeth or the eruption of teeth, sexual maturation is focused on the age of adolescence where there will be changes in the growth of sexual organs, psychomotor such as gross and fine motor movements, bone, each has its time in which they achieve their maximum fullness.This is basically maturation, a succession of events that we must necessarily go through and help us become adults, but what does this have to do with toilet training? It is interesting to mention that the maturation of certain areas has a lot to do with sphincter control, since that is the starting point to determine whether or not the child is ready to begin training. A definition of maturation according to the ABC Definition dictionary (2022): Maturation is a process because it does not happen from one moment to the next, but occurs from the triggering of certain events and elements. In some cases, maturation can last for short periods of time.moments (as, for example, in some insects) while in other living beings it may take years (as, for example, in humans). (p.1).This indicates that it will never happen out of the blue, but that you have to have patience to achieve what you want and be able to develop well, of course whatever happens maturation will happen at some point in our life and will let us know that we are ready to move on to the next stage.We can talk about the child will reach maturation characteristics[4] that will let us know if he/she can start with sphincter control, for this we must take into account that there are external things that can affect the child's maturation and slow it down, such as food that often has to do with the socioeconomic status of the family, the context where he/she develops, the vitamin or nutrients he/she obtained before birth. Among the permissive factors, nutrition, socioeconomic status, the number of children, the affectivity received by the child and the ecological environment in which the child develops as a child. Regarding the psychosocial factors mentioned above, it should be noted that a lack of affectivity in the child's environment decreases growth hormone levels, which return to normal when the child is surrounded by an affective family environment (Olivar & Miranda, 2013, p.37). Then know that absolutely everything that surrounds the child and how it is treated in their family environment will greatly affect their physical growth, development and maturation, also depend on genetic factors and these will have an impact on their evolution, maturation is something innate and can not be changed, but if affected, therefore, the child growing up in a positive environment will have ease for their development and reach all the requirements for a good maturation.The first years of the child will lay the foundations for its growth and development in the future, consequently children in those ages need all the care, proper nutrition, protection and stimulation necessary for their brain to have the development it requires in optimal conditions, in addition to the brain at this age develops at a different speed in which it acquires processes and connections that will not be repeated, therefore, children require special care in early childhood so that their brain can develop properly and achieve the required processes.A child who can start with toilet training shows peculiarities of age, for example: Jumping with both feet, which is a synonym of balance, a language developed enough to warn of the bathroom, that is aware of the need to go to the bathroom, many times when doing their needs in the diaper they hide, because they show embarrassment or ask for privacy by hiding behind an armchair or bed, even entering the bathroom and closing; to learn more about the physiological needs that a child needs to start sphincter control, we will introduce the following topic.

3.1 Physiological Maturation.

When we talk about physiological maturation, this is directed to something more palpable, which can be perceived with the naked eye, which includes physical growth, such as weight gain, height, height, even in food, because as they are in an age of development, they tend to eat more to supply each nutrient needed.The development of the brain has an important point in the physiological maturation, since in the first years of life of the human being is when this is developed in its greater part and at a speed that will not be repeated, specifically the child at this age needs to take care and feed his brain in several ways, giving him the sufficient stimulus to promote a better development, rescuing that the brain does not reach a total maturity, but it acquires an important cerebral development.During the process of brain development, genes and lived experiences-specifically, good nutrition, protection and stimulation through communication, play and responsive caregiver attention-influence neural connections. This combination of innate and acquired lays the foundation for a child's future (UNICEF[5] , 2017,p.1).The importance of the child having a good accompaniment can be crucial for its development, as we can see, it has an important place because it will be the and how you will face in the future, the experiences you have had in the past, and how you will and how they occur will have an impact on the foundations of development that will later affect maturation. Early childhood is the age where changes occur that will have repercussions later on, changes such as language, the beginning of walking, showing interest in certain topics, According to UNICEF, the most valuable pillar is the development of the brain, 80% of which is developed before the age of 3, so that a well-learned toilet training at that stage will result in a good development of the frontal lobe, which helps to control urine, and the nervous system, which gives as an action the stretching of muscles and muscle control, which will result in a good toilet training and makes it considerable to wait for the child to have a correct maturation.Food also has a lot to do, since not having a proper diet is known to bring many problems for the child as tooth decay by eating only junk food or not having a healthy plate of food, taking into account hygiene, of course, obesity that along with food has to do with what the child eats in their day to day, sedentary living in a society blinded by electronic devices such as cell phones or tablets limit movement.Likewise, stunting is a consequence of all the above mentioned, since the body will not get what it needs, so it is a problem with long term repercussions, since the brain will not get the necessary nutrients and will not have the development it needs. problems in the development, maturation of the nervous system and others that will affect not only the palpable but also the internal.For normal functioning of the urinary tract, the autonomic and voluntary nervous systems must be intact, and the muscles of the urinary tract must be functional. Normally, bladder filling stimulates receptors to stretch the bladder and send impulses through the S2 to S4 spinal nerves to the spinal cord and then to the sensory cortex, where the urge to urinate is sensed. A threshold volume, which differs from person to person, triggers awareness of the need to urinate. However, the external urinary sphincter at the bladder outlet is under voluntary control, and generally remains contracted until the person decides to urinate (Shenot & Jefferson, 2020, p.1).As we can see, talking about sphincter control is not only to think about it and it will happen, rather it takes a process that may sound very complicated, but it is rather natural, which will happen without problem or difficulty, besides there are differences between each person and this is important to know, since we can understand that the process with each child will be different, because it will depend on how the person decides to discard, it will be like a signal that begins in the brain and then will have a succession to reach urination.We could argue that brain development has nothing to do with bowel and bladder control, but knowing that the frontal lobe is an important part of the brain's development is a key factor in the development of the brain, and that the frontal lobe is an important part of the brain's development.The development of the process and how each part is connected to be able to perform this action that as adults is already routine, knowing the process makes us aware of how for a child it can be difficult to assimilate what will happen and how to achieve it, so it is important that the companion knows what happens in the body to perform the action of defecation and urination. The companion will know what is happening or will have some knowledge, therefore, will be more careful to be the person who will support the child; recognizing that maturity is to reach the maximum point of development that the body needs and through this the body to function properly and specifically better than before, is a crucial point for the human being, because through physiological maturation will have a better future, so to speak because remember that the maturation has an impact for what will come of the child. On the other hand, knowing what affects the physiological maturity of the human being is important, because it will depend on the influence received or received in their environment, talking about the family environment, cultural, socioeconomic, will be relevant points to forge the child and what will leave its mark on its growth, in its maturity of the nervous system, so anyone who has a relationship with the child will be important to emphasize the responsibility of being a good influence for the child, and help stimulate it to achieve what is required.In the early childhood stage, the brain goes through something called plasticity, named after the author William James, referring to the fact that it acquires skills and can change, therefore, the functioning can differ, the nervous system can adapt depending on what the child needs.The companion should help to ensure that this plasticity does not diminish, but rather stimulate the brain system so that it can learn more quickly, so that if we stimulate the child to achieve sphincter control, learning will be much better. Emphasizing that we will not do everything for him, but, on the contrary, we will give him the tools to be able to achieve it by himself, making him know and experience by himself his learning capacity, a fact is that the body works in an incredible way consequently it is not right to rush, rather it defers us to be able to achieve the functioning he needs by himself, letting every necessary characteristic flow.The physiological maturity also includes the development of balance, which in the sphincter control is one of the most important pillars, because through this we will know if the child can already perform actions such as taking down clothes alone, sit on the toilet or potty. The balance is how the child achieves a cohesion of all the senses for the proper functioning, this as all I know should be trained and stimulated to achieve good development, having well developed balance, the child will more easily do activities such as reading, writing, toilet training, and so on.The sense of balance is the name given to the sensations of equilibrium, that is, the spatial orientation and regulation of balance in space caused by this sensory system, among which are the vestibular receptors (hearing), the proprioceptive receptors of the skeletal musculature and joints, as well as the skin receptors.

These are interconnected in the brainstem and cerebral cortical areas with the visual structures, including the nuclei that control the ocular musculature, the auditory pathway and the reflex center of the cerebellum (Andersson, 2015, p.1).Balance is a fundamental part for the child to be able to move freely, giving as a reference that he can already perform articulated movements more easily, it will no longer be like at the beginning, he can stumble constantly, he does not hold his legs or head, he goes sideways, rather it will be a more controlled movement, therefore, it will give us as an indication that he can already jump with both feet which means that he can control the muscles of the lower part of his body, therefore he can control his sphincter, which is a muscle, remembering that it is a muscle. At the age where sphincter control begins, a series of changes also begins in the child's body, such as increase in body mass, increase in height, weight gain, which is linked to the natural growth of the child, also changes occur in their character, emotions and begin "the terrible twos" where there are plenty of tantrums in children, but if we can think they are changes in their physiology that can be disturbing in them and need to get it out somehow, because they still do not fully understand what is happening. All these changes can be bought with puberty where the change goes from child to adolescent, in this case the change is from baby to toddler, therefore, they stop doing things they did before, they can achieve things they did before, they can achieve things they did before, they can achieve things they did before, they can achieve things they did before, they can achieve things they did before, they can achieve things they did before.before not, the changes are not only physical but also cognitive such as interest in new objects, exploring colors and shapes, psychological such as fear of new people or the unknown, understanding that they are not one with their mother but an individual, etc. Consequently, they need to be supported and understood. We will also learn about cognitive maturation, which will help them acquire certain skills that will help them in the future and which is very important for toilet training.

3.2 Cognitive maturation.

Cognitive maturation tells us about the knowledge that we acquire depending on our growth and reasoning capacity, this maturation begins when we are born, because we begin to understand how the world works, what surrounds us in essence, also begins to increase in childhood and adolescence, we can say that the child can begin to recognize how your body works knowing that it is a somewhat complex process, externalize that the movements take orders from the brain and through a joint work of organs, muscles and therefore begins to have the ability to control certain movements or actions.The author Jean Piaget talks about this topic in his theories of cognitive development, where we can know that the sensory-motor stages, pre-operational, concrete operations and formal operations tell us about different stages of the human being, where what the child experiences will form his knowledge or ideas of what happens in what surrounds him, also from the experiences, the child will be able to assimilate if the experience helped him/her to achieve something and the accommodation to know when to use that knowledge.Specifically, the appearance of language is an indication that the child is beginning to reason, albeit with certain limitations. Thus, it can be said that cognitive development in early childhood is free and imaginative, but through its constant use, the mental understanding of the world improves more and more (CAMPO, 2009, p.342).In this way, language becomes an indication of what the child is learning and what he/she is surrounded by, in addition to the fact that cognitive maturity will be achieved in a free way, but the author emphasizes that the development of maturity must be supported through stimulation, especially in what surrounds and the experiences that the child will have.The child at the beginning of his cognitive maturity will be the determinant of what he learns and if it will serve him in his growth, the child will have the ability to help his own cognitive maturity that specifically has a significant growth in childhood, adolescence, but it is in adulthood when the human being manages to reach one hundred percent; this maturity is intended that the child builds his knowledge, then starting with the training of sphincter control will make the child have experiences of how it happens.In this way, the experience and knowledge he has had will be decisive and will serve him in the future for his development; here the importance is that if the correct stimulation is provided, the child will know that the experience he has had will serve him for his future development. To this end, cognitive maturation plays an important role in the development of sphincter control, as it will be the basis for what the child experiences during training and whether he/she manages to have control in a positive or negative way.According to the Universidad Pedagógica Nacional - Hidalgo (1999):Developmental psychology has shown that, from the acquisition of oral language to the culmination of concrete operations, the period between two and six years of age is dominated by the symbolic function whose basic manifestations are drawing, play and verbal language. (P.264).In this sense we can know that the child will learn based on play and what he can develop based on this, how language, play and drawing are correlated for the child and how they are used in each activity, these elements will be pillars of what the child will develop and how he will form his maturity and development.Cognitive maturity encompasses what is adaptation, because the brain seeks ways to know what is happening, assimilate it, and then reproduce it already learned, or imitate what he saw, since in the age of 2 to 3 years are at the stage where they learn by imitation also making this a special feature in toilet training, by the fact that if you can imitate the movements of someone else will be easier to achieve control. Cognitive maturation can have special characteristics such as the child can solve problems using exploration, curiosity and observation, which will lead him to something he already saw or knows to solve his problem, using what he already knew and how he saw it applied or how he applied it, because he will already have the knowledge of how it is done and what reaction it has, this coupled with trial and error, since he will have no problem with failure, because his curiosity is greater to know what will happen.The child will interrelate with the environment at the beginning through the perceptual and motor manipulation of objects, this will serve to obtain information, recognize, remember and above all act materially on the environment, at this time intelligence is of a practical nature.

The evolution of intelligence in the infant, its interaction with the physical world and object permanence has been contrasted by different authors who have verified a similar sequence (Faas, 2018, p. 203). At the beginning, cognitive maturity will always depend on what surrounds the child and in this way he will build it, and later, having as a base what he has already learned or experienced thanks to the stimulation that was given to him from the outside, he will then have an increase in intelligence based on play, language, and drawing, which are a fundamental part of a child's development.Likewise, the senses are an important part of what is cognitive maturation, because it is through them that the body receives these signals of certain stimuli, which creates the need for a solution to a situation or problem, which will make the child have the need to experiment. to get an answer, this will enable you to activate your cognition to understand what is happening or will happen. The child begins to understand what is happening in the moment, what can happen in the present, thanks to the process of conceptualization of objects, shapes, situations, activities, etc.; it is important to use communication at their level so that they can express themselves correctly, at the beginning symbols can be used, so that they can represent what they need, such as people, places, activities, this can stimulate their cognitive maturity and seek more to learn. The child understands his point of view as the only one that exists. He is learning that the identity of objects can be permanent even if their external appearance is modified, as well as the **causality** of some actions, although not in a reversible way (things can only happen in a certain way and in a certain sense) (Cuídate plus, 2015, p.1). (Cuídate plus, 2015, p.1).Then the child not only reasons on what he sees, but already asks himself questions about what happens and what he should do, already begins to have a behavior of the self as a whole and a first, knowing that, although there are around him individual of the same value, his egocentrism does not make him see beyond and his cognition makes him believe that it is right to think about himself and no one else.Cognitive maturity is intimately related to sphincter control, so that the child will take his first experience with the This will determine whether the child reproduces in a positive way what he has learned, because thanks to this information he will have tools to execute the same task, he will then be able to codify his conduct and have actions for his behavior.An example of this would be when the child who had a bad teaching will try to hold back as much as possible to avoid going to the bathroom, soiling his underwear hiding for fear of retaliation, he will have constipation problems, because his bad experience will make him know what will come and will not want to face the consequences, otherwise when the child has learned in a positive way he will know that he can freely ask for support, go to the toilet without problem, make or warn at any time.According to the social cognitive current "observing models does not guarantee learning or the ability to later exhibit the behaviors, but it fulfills information and motivational functions: it communicates the probability of the consequences of the acts and modifies the degree of motivation of the observers to act in the same way." (Faas, 2018, p.68).Cognitive maturity is then built by the child, it is not that it is transmitted, but the child builds it according to experiences and motivation or stimulation that is given to him, because, he will take as an impulse what he could already know or see and from there he will know what he can achieve and how to do it, cognition is the result of what was experienced, what he learned to imitate, imagination, games, language, using each one for the benefit of his knowledge and development. Cognitive maturation has and will always have a very important place in the life of a child, since thanks to this we can know what is beneficial and what is not, in addition to clarifying doubts about the reason why it is linked to toilet training, because we can know that once again it is proven that how he learns or how he has the example will affect the attitudes and actions he takes in the future or rather how he uses that information for his own benefit. Likewise, we can learn about a topic linked to the previous ones, this topic helps us to know what a child must fulfill in social maturity to have enough tools for the beginning of the training.

3.3 Social maturation

The social process helps the human being to integrate into a community having as a basis appropriate behaviors to be able to correlate with their environment, which comes from their relationship at home with the people around the child, knowing that any example that has imitates it, therefore, the pillar of the home should be respect for the child to have a favorable behavior in their social environment, in this way can show ability to be autonomous, as it should project how he learned to relate.Every human being is born with a personality that makes him have contact with his environment, with time his family nucleus will make him take his place in society, but it is thanks to this that the child structures his position and relationship with the external world, being the first socialization the most important; a good level of socialization is the most important one. developmental, physical and emotional development will make the individual socially responsible and mature.When the child is born and during its growth, experiential processes begin that help the child to relate to the outside world, the child in its understanding will begin to feel a crucial part of a group, because its family context will make it feel this way, to later integrate into a larger group when it begins its preschool years, in these years how it was influenced will have great repercussions, because the attachment, the relationship with parents, etc. will have a very important role for its social development.In relation to the theories that explain how social knowledge is formed, some authors, such as Moscovici, postulate that living in society the person incorporates the representations of the social group to which he or she belongs. For others, such as Piaget, social knowledge is constructed by subjects through an interaction between their cognitive capacities and their participation in social life. For Vigotsky, individual development and social processes are intimately linked, all functions originate as relationships between human beings (Faas, 2018, p. 392).The authors Moscovici, Piaget and Vigotsky, can tell us about what affects the child in their social development and how it will be projected during their growth, making each element crucial to be socially mature and develop with welfare, encompassing every interaction that has with the outside will affect the decisions and actions that the child takes; similarly will affect the social group to which he/she belongs, e.g., way of acting, permitted and forbidden patterns for him/her.The child acquires social skills specific to his context in the daily interaction he has with the people around him, for example, when he begins with social characteristics such as smiling, body language with people, even forms of courtesy of his culture, as mentioned before, learning by observation will have greater weight.The socialization process is closely related to what the child acquires, behavior, depends on how he learns from others, as he grows and matures, he will have the ability to accept responsibilities and act coherently "In this way, Vigotsky considers that learning stimulates and activates a variety of mental processes that emerge in the framework of interaction with other people, interaction that occurs in various contexts and is always mediated by language"(Faas, 2018, p.74). In this sense, language also forms a very important part for social maturity. If children learn in a positive way to develop socially, they will be able to control and regulate their emotions, because they will take into account that they are responsible for what they can cause and affect; socialization allows the child to acquire knowledge, attitudes, skills that will serve to develop in society, today we can see that there are different factors that influence the socialization of children, because in a modern world not only the family will be a conduit to shape their behavior, but social networks take a very strong role in influencing children.Television and all existing platforms can play a relevant role in the socialization process and thus help in a negative way, since the screens, in addition to affecting the eyesight, affect a level where the child has no interest in experiential learning, which will affect their cognition and therefore their socialization, because by only looking for answers on the internet or other platforms they will no longer have any interaction with the outside world and will not form emotional ties with other people.Socialization has an important weight in the child's personality, because external agents will be the ones that form his personality, he will also learn to know the characteristics of his environment or culture, socialization also has to do with stimuli, because it will be based on these that social maturity can be given or he can develop and form his own perception of society, thanks to this the child will adapt to the culture and society in which he lived.During the age in which sphincter control training can begin, the child begins to have an external socialization, as it will no longer depend only on the parents, as it will take decisive parts for their socialization of those around him starting to have contact with other children of their age or that may mean a change in their daily lives, understanding that the child is no longer only forged based on the parents, they must take care of the integrity and self-esteem of the child, as very sensitive children can be damaged at a critical level by their social environment.Likewise, parents must understand that the security with which they forge their child will depend on them, knowing that the age of egocentrism begins, speaking that the child will think of himself as a whole, therefore, it may be difficult for them to accept the opinion of others or their point of view, as they always seek to be the center of attention, "The socialization process demands the internalization of an accumulation of values and a procedure of symbols that are transformed into language that only with maturity will be able to be expressed and articulated, the infant begins to relate what he does, to point out what he is going to do" (Del castillo, 2017 p. 20). Socialization then encompasses a whole as what was taught at home, what society will forge in the child and how he/she will internalize it.Some characteristics of social maturity in children may be that they begin to consider the consequences of any act or comment they make, they begin to distinguish themselves from others as individuals, they recognize what surrounds them and can comment on it, they have a good language to be able to develop, they begin to recognize the things that are good and bad, so they can make their own decisions, they can have ideas not for their own benefit but a benefit as a whole that helps to improve as a society or person, this happens little by little but with greater credibility for a child.In conclusion, social maturation will occur based on external stimuli that influence the child, starting with the family, therefore, toilet training will begin to occur when the child is socially apt or has the characteristics already mentioned, as this will indicate that the child has sufficient autonomy, which will help you focus on the basis of the support and need you have.

3.4 Adaptive maturation.

Adaptive maturation for the child that begins with sphincter control is important, since it can be taken as the integral condition of the child, that is, what the child has already developed as skills that he/she uses on a daily basis, for example, changing clothes, eating alone, going to the bathroom alone, etc. Therefore, we can see that for sphincter control it is necessary for the child to be able to perform these tasks on his/her own to demonstrate his/her autonomy, confidence and control.Adaptive maturity leads children to begin to make their own decisions and actions during their day, in particular to seek independence from their parents, caregivers or attachment figures, as they begin to know that they are capable of performing tasks on their own and begin to see themselves as big children who no longer require help to do things, but rather demand their autonomy to be able to act on their own.Adapting can be taken to mean that they no longer need support, but it is important to let them know that they must place themselves in a balance where they can act alone, but not without control. "In this process of internalization, the child accepts as his own social standards of behavior fundamental for socialization and achieve to develop self-control of behavior to adapt to assimilated social expectations in what is known as self-regulation" (Campo, 2011, p.96). Therefore, the child must know his or her The process of self-regulating one's actions and knowing the consequences begins.When we talk about adaptive maturity we can say that the child has managed to develop skills appropriate to his age, so that in this way he can make them functional to experience day by day what is demanded in his environment; during the child's development he will show that he can understand certain situations by placing the attention he can take in these, to have responsibility and understand what happens, in addition to performing actions that are useful to him such as having personal hygiene, to be able to feed himself.The adaptive process from a baby to a young child has also the importance of how the child perceives himself, when he starts to have a notion of himself as someone capable, this will make his unconscious let him know that he is doing well, therefore, it makes him get security, then this influences his social development and his personality, adaptation will always bring different or difficult situations for a child's life, as he will try that he can attach every skill and behavior with which he was prepared at home.Knowing how to behave and apply the knowledge already acquired helps to be part of what it is to adapt to a society, to a community, because he will do what he thinks is right; the human being acquires changes during his growth, emotional, biological, cognitive, behavioral changes, which help him to grow in his development and adaptation to the outside world. These changes will help to face both their needs and external needs, emphasizing that both the internal and external influences the child's life, we can understand that in order to generate adaptive maturation the child must have certain characteristics to know that he is ready, some characteristics are: to know that their actions have a consequence, to have sufficient skills to cope in their environment, to have skills acquired by experimentation with their context.Adaptive maturity encompasses skills that the child must develop having contact with his environment, which will help him to be part of a society; an example of what he needs is the development of language, thinking, his coordination, qualities that are expected to reach one hundred percent so that the development of childhood is enriching for the child and is of fundamental support to know how to react in his daily life, being these tools for daily situations.

3.5 What the experts think.

The topic of sphincter control has as arguments several theories of important authors for early childhood, authors such as Piaget, Freud, Montessori, Erickson are some of which we can take arguments and stages on which to base the development of the child and has much to do with toilet training, which emphasize that the maturation is unique to each body, not rushed, rather the adult plays the role of being a companion that encourages and stimulates the child to reach its mission.

Piaget	Freud	Montessori	Erickson
2 to 7 years	18 months 3 years	0 to 6 years	2 to 4 years
Theory of cognitive development.	Psychoanalysis and psychosexual theory.	Theory of autonomous learning.	Theory of psychosocial development.
Pre-operational stage	Anal stage	Childhood	Autonomy vs. embarrassment stage
During this stage the child does not yet conceive certain characteristics that make him/her an individual aware of what is going on outside, as he/she is not yet able to understand every piece of information one hundred percent. Therefore, the control of sphincters can become disturbing if not is explained from easy for him.	Sensitivity is directed to defecation, being vital sphincter control and an important part of this stage, because it will begin to have different sensations; it knows the pleasure through cleanliness and feels good. with himself in the satisfaction of his mother for her achievements in the control.	Learning is entirely constructed by the child, the adult represents only a support and accompaniment, it is crucial to emphasize that the adult should not intervene to do it for the child, but only for the child. observes and indicates the to do, emphasizes that a little help can ruin the child's progress.	Hygienic learning is vital for the child to reach his autonomy, he receives guidance from others, but the activities are done by him alone, a balance between shame and self-confidence must be worked out. to reach the confidence in the itself; the control sphincter will help the child to develop the difference between let go and hold on to something.

Table 1: Authors of development theories (2022, Morales).

Sphincter control is a very important issue for children, the reality is that it is not known one hundred percent or why we should wait, the interest is in knowing what is behind the control and how we can support as adults to a child who begins with this process, how not to lose patience, understand that we should not wait just because, rather know what processes and characteristics the child must meet to start with the training.In conclusion, the child must go through processes that are very important for its development, knowing what to achieve will make us understand that toilet training must take maturity processes that the body itself reaches at its own pace, many times we only hear it is not yet time to learn, but we do not know what is behind everything the child needs to start with the training, knowing what differentiates the development of the child from the rest of the body. maturity, the cognitive maturity that a child must have or reach at an early age, physical maturity, adaptive maturity, etc., are fields that must be covered so that the child can achieve complete control without any lacking.

CHAPTER 4

CORRECT STEPS FOR SPHINCTER CONTROL ACCOMPANIMENT.

We often give children answers to remember instead of problems to be solved.
-Roger Lewin.

As we already know, sphincter control has a series of processes and unique characteristics to start with the training, the accompaniment as parents or teachers must be full of patience, confidence and knowledge of the subject, which is the most important of all so that we can understand what the child goes through to control and what is the famous saying "not yet ready" but go beyond to know how it should mature to understand why it takes time to learn it a hundred percent.The child has countless questions about how the world works, what surrounds him/her, how he/she is used, the adult must answer those questions and be a crucial and safe support for the child to know that he/she is learning and feel complete in the enriching environment that the parent must provide, this alludes to the sphincter control, since the parents will be the beginning and impulse for the security that the child feels when learning about the subject from the people he/she trusts the most, which will be the pillar of future learning.The positive parenting style reproves any incorrect behavior that stops the child's learning, violent behavior, discriminatory behavior that makes the child doubt and feel insecure about the decisions or activities that he/she will carry out, therefore Therefore, the current seeks to enrich the child's knowledge with good manners and having respect as the main indicative; the activities are always guided but not carried out by adults in order to improve the child's autonomy and self-confidence.Some correct steps to foster both autonomy, self-esteem, learning for the child are as follows: Let him act alone, so that he makes mistakes, but learns from them.Give the child physical space, in this way the child will understand that he/she can do things by him/herself and not necessarily depend on someone else. Let him think so he can learn to recognize good decisions and solve problems on his own.Do not be discouraged by attitudes such as "you will never succeed", impatience, impatience, impatience that because you want to learn quickly, you do not know support but pressure. Teach them to look for answers or solutions by providing accompaniment such as finding a book that talks about the topic, a video, a song that motivates them.Remind him that he is not alone, as a responsible adult he should be accompanied, given his space, but not neglected so that he can feel safe in his environment.During this process the routine is a very good way to establish play and toileting times, so that the child begins to get used to the toilet visit.If the child is afraid, cries, is insecure, he/she should be respected and not be forced to do the activity, on the contrary, you should wait so that by example he/she sees that it is safe and wait until he/she is interested.It is extremely important to motivate the child with actions such as encouragement, praise, but not exaggerated, as it can be counterproductive, but it will always be nice to let him/her know that he/she is doing something in a correct way.Research application.

The research was applied with four children who are in the age to begin sphincter control, taking into account that they meet the essential characteristics for the beginning, during the research we will focus on observing the behavior during training, having the guide as the main support for us to know what actions to take, we will take into account the attention that parents took to accompany the children, actions taken in children who already control sphincters in the day care center "love and fantasy" where surveys were taken from parents and teachers.

4.1 Questions and answers.

For the creation of the guide we conducted surveys to parents who have children who are already 100% potty trained (see Annex A) and teachers, asking what methods they used, calculating ages for the beginning and some tactics or tips, in order to know what areas we will be working on and what we will be working on in the future (see Annex B). that we must know to start with the guide that will be of help to parents who are beginning to train sphincter control.

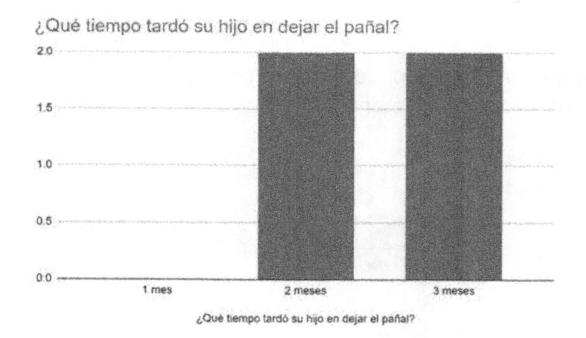

¿Qué tiempo tardó su hijo en dejar el pañal?

We can observe that 100% of 2 to 3 months is the age, it is the time it takes for them to leave the diaper.

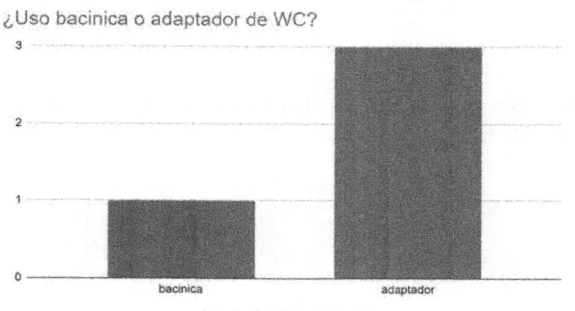

¿Uso bacinica o adaptador de WC?

43

As we can see the use of the potty is not indispensable for the practice of the training, since this goes in the toilet and will make it easier to make the child lose the fear, according to the comment of the teachers, the potty is more complicated because it is necessary to move from a potty to a larger toilet, which can be disturbing to the child.

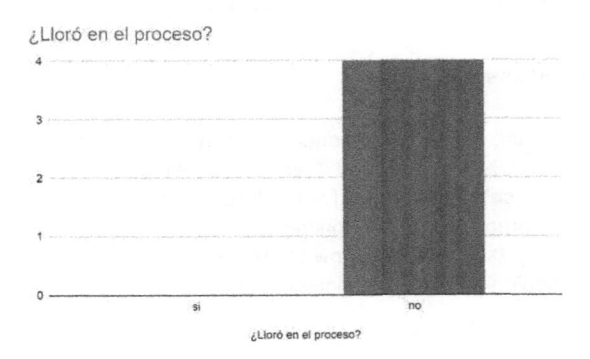

¿Lloró en el proceso?

si	no
0	4

The anguish of the child crying or suffering is important for the parents, but you may think that it will pass, but it is different.

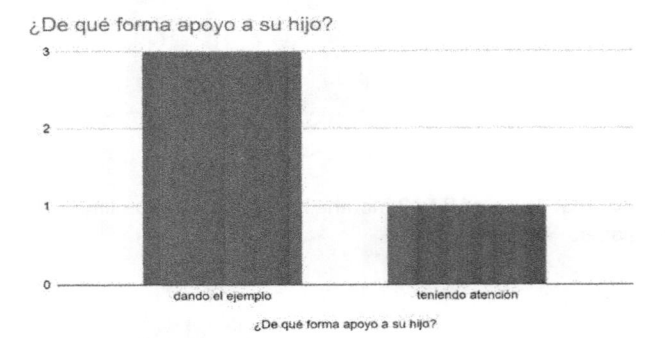

¿De qué forma apoyo a su hijo?

dando el ejemplo	teniendo atención
3	1

The parents, seeing that the child imitates everything he sees, proceed to take this point as a key to training.

¿Qué edad tenía cuando comenzó con el proceso?

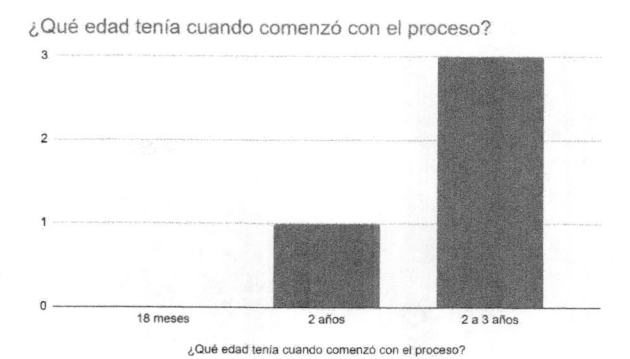

The average age at which parents started with the training is 2 to 3 years old, which you might think they started big, but as we could see above, children are the ones who show when they already start.

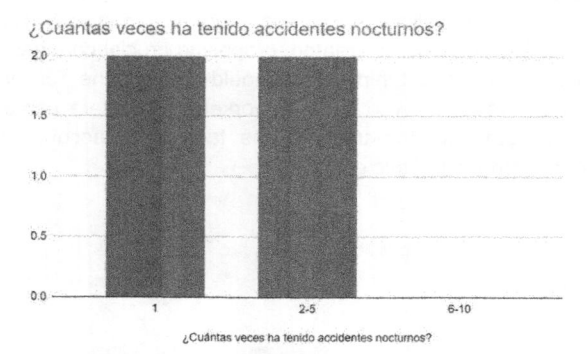

¿Cuántas veces ha tenido accidentes nocturnos?

Nocturnal accidents are totally normal at the beginning of the child's training, it is important to be patient at this stage.

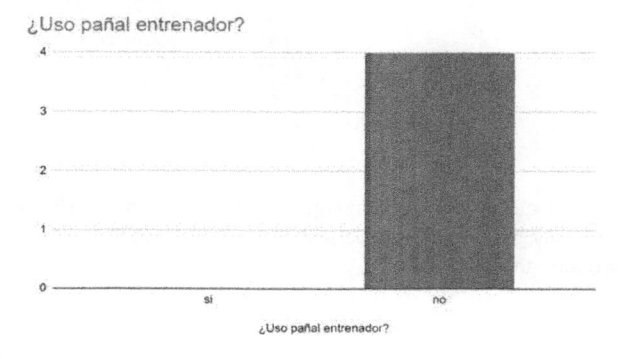

¿Uso pañal entrenador?

The use of the trainer diaper as we can see is not relevant and nothing happens if it is not used.

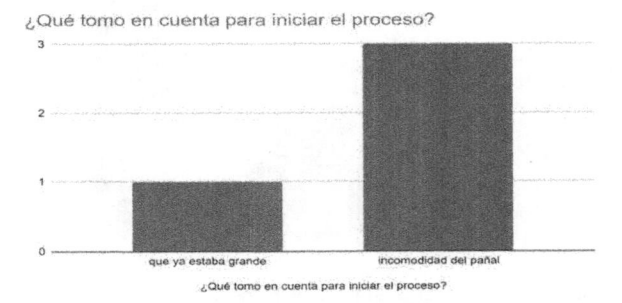

¿Qué tomo en cuenta para iniciar el proceso?

In the beginning of the training for these parents it was important to see what they were already uncomfortable with and age was important as well. As could be observed, the parents who were surveyed commented that their children started at an appropriate age for physical, social and emotional maturity. Taking this into account, the guide for parents was created, proposing crucial changes in the infants' routine, also taking into account things that should not be done; for this, the opinion of 5 educators (see Annex B) who work or worked in day care centers where it is more common to start with the training was taken into account, with valuable contributions for the creation of this guide.

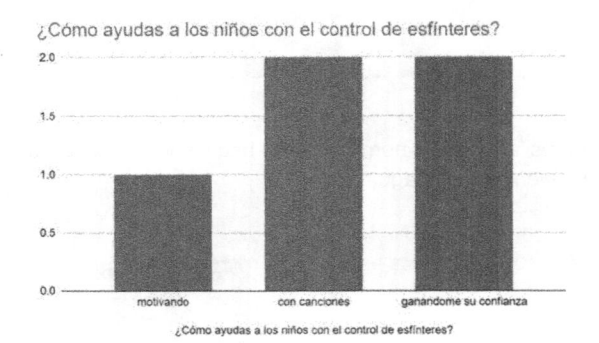

¿Cómo ayudas a los niños con el control de esfínteres?

The role of the educator during the training is fundamental, since she is the one who follows up the training or gives the beginning, we can see that the songs and the motivations are fundamental.

¿Cuál es el método o métodos que has usado?

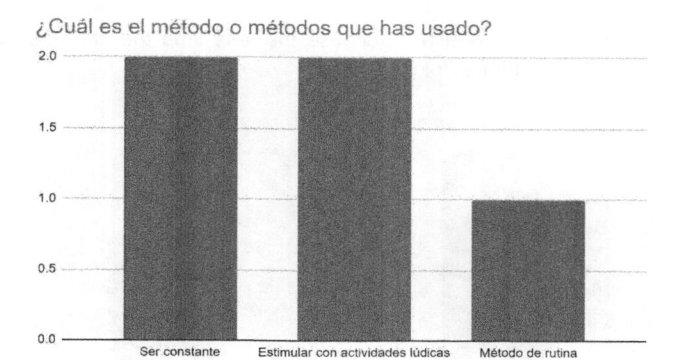

The experience is crucial to know what educators can share and take it as a reference.

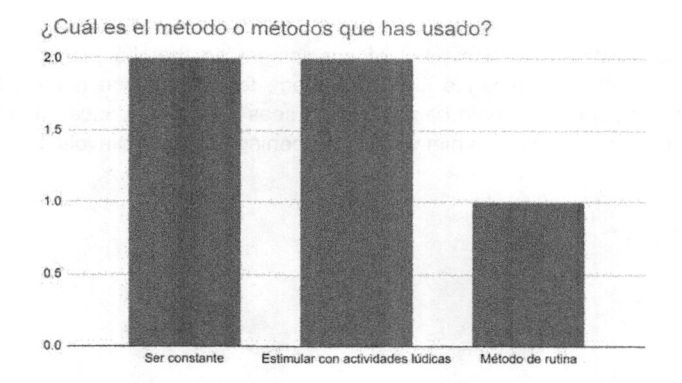

¿Cuál es el método o métodos que has usado?

As we can see, educators can use different training methods to make learning more enjoyable.

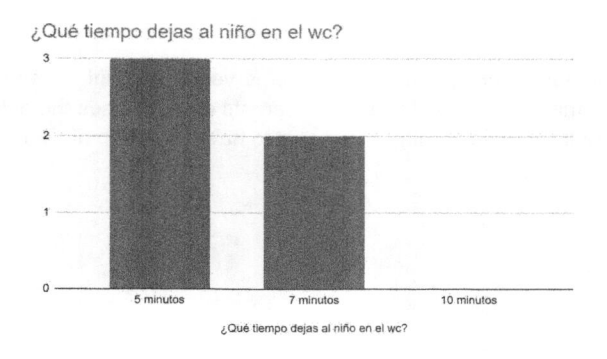

¿Qué tiempo dejas al niño en el wc?

The time the child is left is relevant because the less time the child spends in the W.C. stays, the child is better employed.

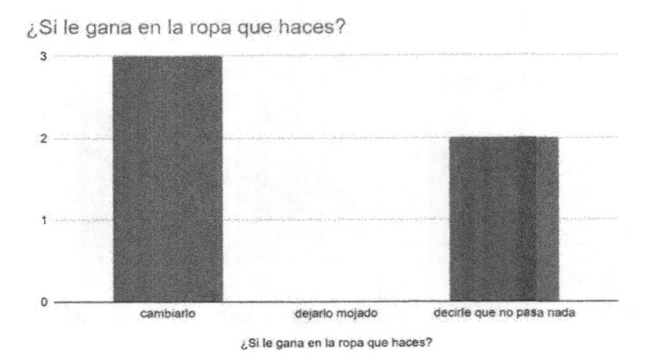

¿Si le gana en la ropa que haces?

cambiarlo	dejarlo mojado	decirle que no pasa nada
3	0	2

¿Si le gana en la ropa que haces?

Leaving the child wet as a symbol of punishment so that he learns faster is a reprehensible act that damages his self-esteem; telling him that nothing happens makes the child not try to hold back since he sees no consequence, therefore, the best thing to do is to explain to him what is happening and how to avoid it.

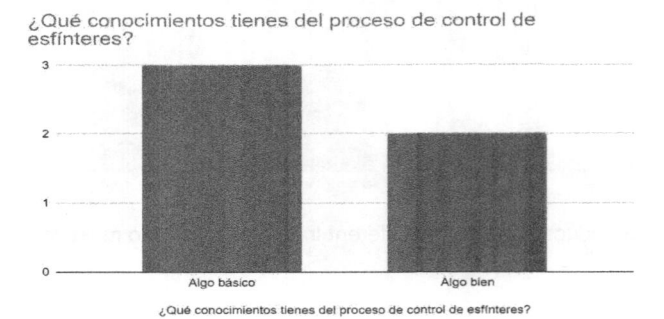

¿Qué conocimientos tienes del proceso de control de esfínteres?

Algo básico	Algo bien
3	2

¿Qué conocimientos tienes del proceso de control de esfínteres?

Having a basis for initiating sphincter control is very important for educators, since they are the primary help in addition to the parents or sometimes the only support for the child for control, consequently, it is crucial to have a backup of what to do.

¿Usas adaptador o bacinica en tu empleo?

adaptador	bacinica	wc
3	1	1

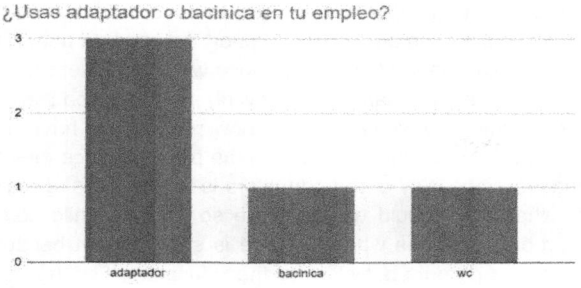

¿Usas adaptador o bacinica en tu empleo?

As we can see the use of the adaptor is better in the training practice, since it goes in the toilet and will make it easier to make the child lose the fear, according to the teacher's comment, the potty is more complicated. because it is necessary to move from a potty to a larger toilet, which may disturb the child.

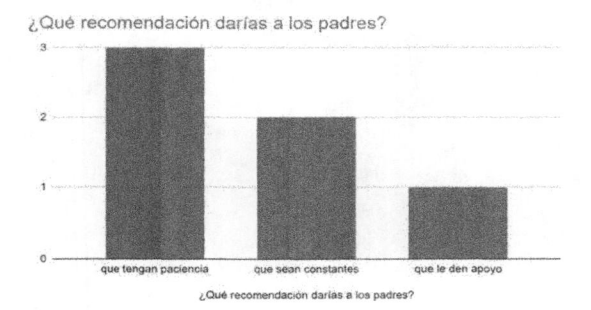

¿Qué recomendación darías a los padres?

que tengan paciencia	que sean constantes	que le den apoyo
3	2	1

¿Qué recomendación darías a los padres?

Noting what the parent should do is to be a supportive figure, patience, constancy, never do things for the child.

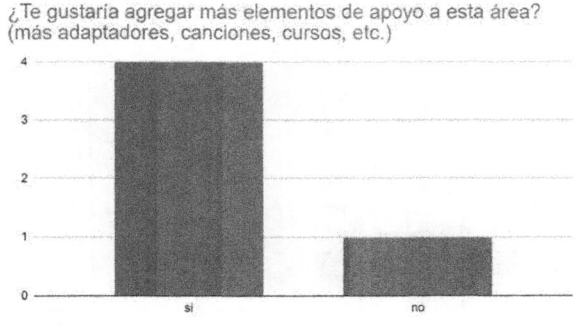

¿Te gustaría agregar más elementos de apoyo a esta área? (más adaptadores, canciones, cursos, etc.)

si	no
4	1

¿Te gustaría agregar más elementos de apoyo a esta área? (más adaptadores, canciones, cursos...)

It is very important that the directors or heads of each institution employ their educators well so that they can provide the support the children need.They also need to do it with previous knowledge, since ignorance will cause them to make mistakes that affect the child.The importance of knowing how the teachers think is very valuable because in this way we can get to know people who have a bond with the child, but most of them have little support from the parents, since they think that they should do all the work, the duty of the educators is to support and make the parents responsible for what they should use at home so that the child comes out of the diaper without problems, this is why the guide is so important because it will be a support mainly for the parents but also for the educators. For the beginning of the application of the guide, we took into account what the children could achieve, the parents answered a survey (see Annex C) to know if it is time to start with the guide or wait a little to achieve progress without affecting the child, on this it was decided whether to share the guide to start with the training.

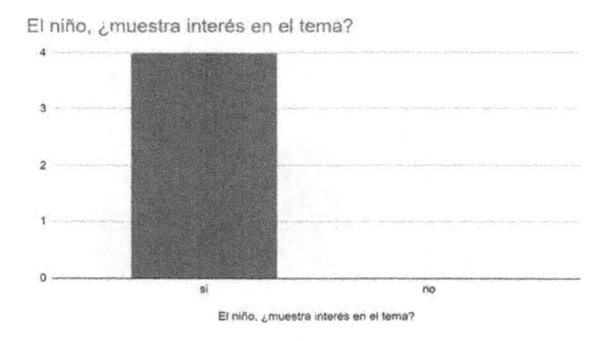

El niño, ¿muestra interés en el tema?

It is important to note that the child has an interest or else he/she will be forced to start and this will have repercussions later on.

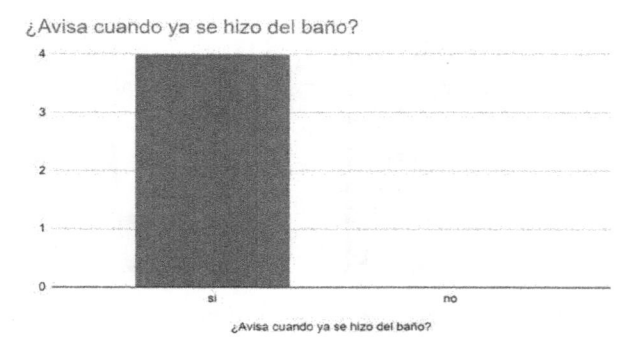

¿Avisa cuando ya se hizo del baño?

As we can see, the fact that the child notifies is crucial to know that he/she is starting to be ready, since in this way he/she seeks to communicate what he/she feels; at the beginning it will be with signs, but the stimulus must be given to support him/her in the language so that he/she can notify.

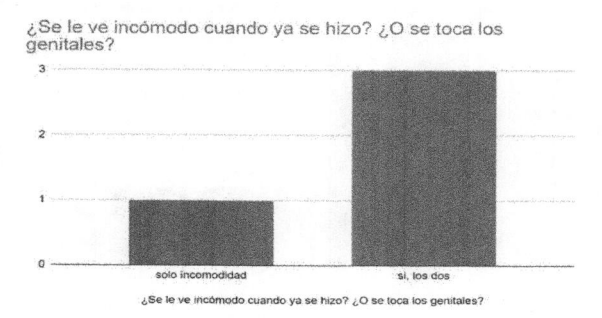

¿Se le ve incómodo cuando ya se hizo? ¿O se toca los genitales?

Another key point to start with training is that it begins with discomfort.

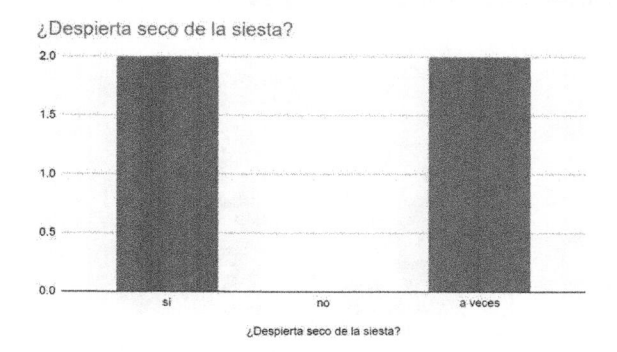

¿Despierta seco de la siesta?

Dryness is a sign that the child is beginning to control the sphincter for shorter periods of time.

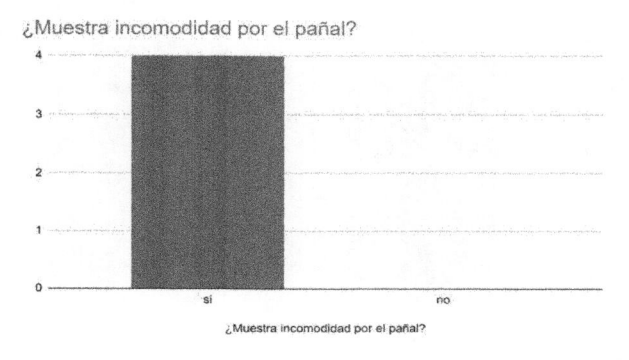

¿Muestra incomodidad por el pañal?

Having discomfort when feeling the waste is different from the child feeling discomfort all the time the diaper is on, therefore, when the child feels discomfort all the time it is crucial to start training.

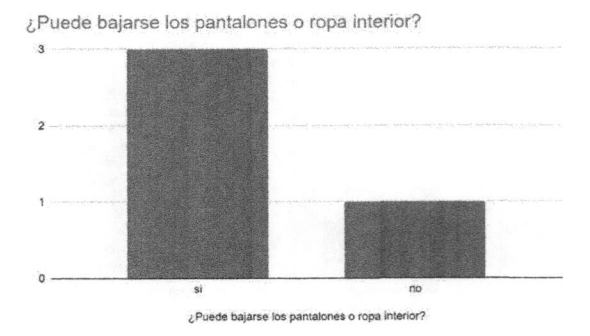

¿Puede bajarse los pantalones o ropa interior?

	si	no
	3	1

¿Puede bajarse los pantalones o ropa interior?

Generating autonomy in the child is important, for this we must begin to know if the child has certain skills to perform simple activities.

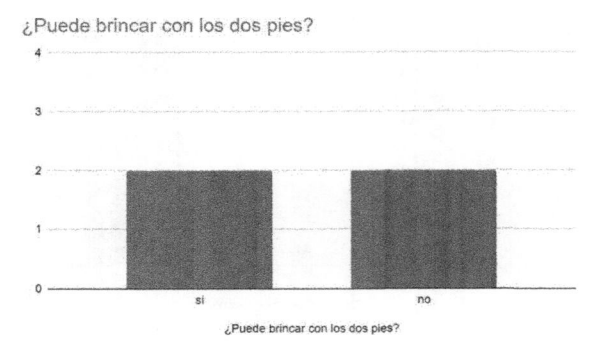

¿Puede brincar con los dos pies?

	si	no
	2	2

¿Puede brincar con los dos pies?

Knowing if the child has control over the lower part of his body is relevant because this is where he will exercise the sphincter and thus be able to control it.

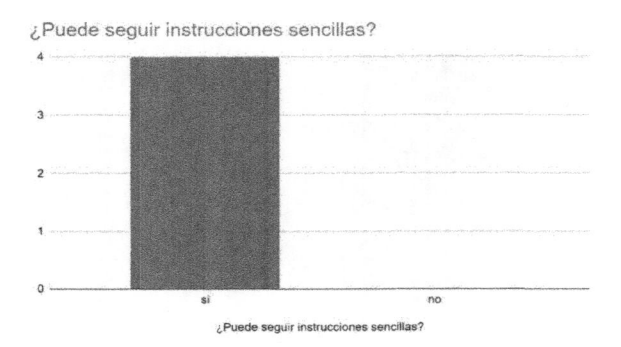

¿Puede seguir instrucciones sencillas?

	si	no
	4	0

¿Puede seguir instrucciones sencillas?

The child being able to follow simple instructions will help so that the parent is not a doer, but rather just a companion who guides the training.

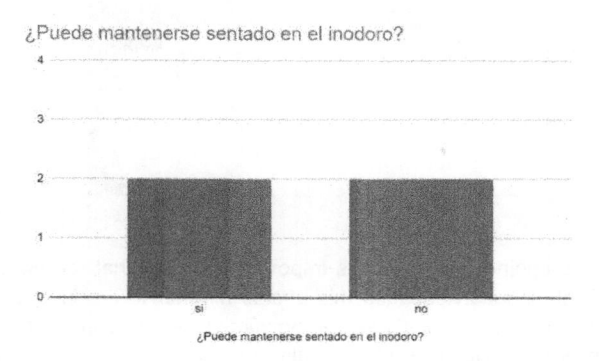

¿Puede mantenerse sentado en el inodoro?

	si	no
	2	2

¿Puede mantenerse sentado en el inodoro?

Fear can affect the child to the level of trauma or generate a bad experience, therefore, you should start by knowing if he/she can be in contact with the W.C. or wait for him/her to become familiar with it.

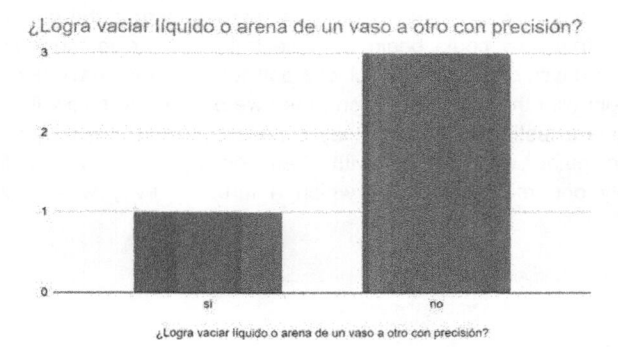

¿Logra vaciar líquido o arena de un vaso a otro con precisión?

	si	no
	1	3

¿Logra vaciar líquido o arena de un vaso a otro con precisión?

Balance and coordination are a crucial part to start with the training, since they will be used during their stay in the bathroom, being able to perform actions like this will let the child know that he/she is able to perform complicated actions.

¿En casa hay alguna situación que le esté afectando como: el nacimiento de un hermanito, cambio de casa; muerte de un s...

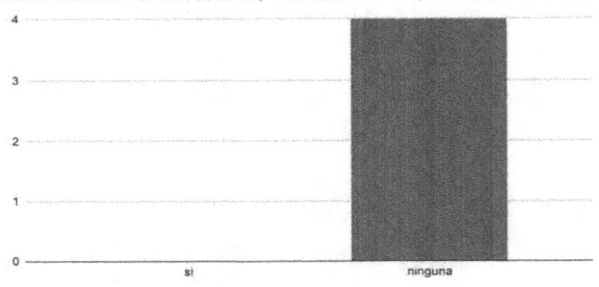

[Bar chart: "si" = 0, "ninguna" = 4]

To start with the sphincter control it is important to know that the child is not going through a difficult situation because this affects him/her to the level that he/she will not be able to advance or will have a significant setback, since the control also depends on how the child is psychologically.Having parental support and interest is crucial, for the fact that we can trust that it will not be a job of one person, but of a set that will make accompaniment in a positive way, resulting in a short training, which will help the child in his autonomy, self-esteem, control of his body; the sharing of guidance as a backup will be proof of how prior knowledge can achieve things successfully.Taking into account what the parents responded, the guide was shared with them so that they could begin with the training, or else they were asked to support the child with stimulation to achieve activities that they have not yet mastered and thus begin with the accompaniment, they were asked to follow the steps of the guide and give a testimony of what they experienced and how they felt during the process, the guide was shared with them on May 15 to ask for progress approximately one month later, for which a further survey was conducted (see AnnexC).

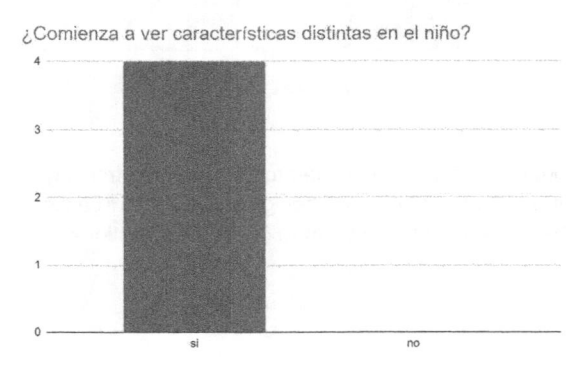

¿Comienza a ver características distintas en el niño?

[Bar chart: "si" = 4, "no" = 0]

The characteristics of the children will change according to the different activities that they are given as a routine.

¿Cómo cuál?

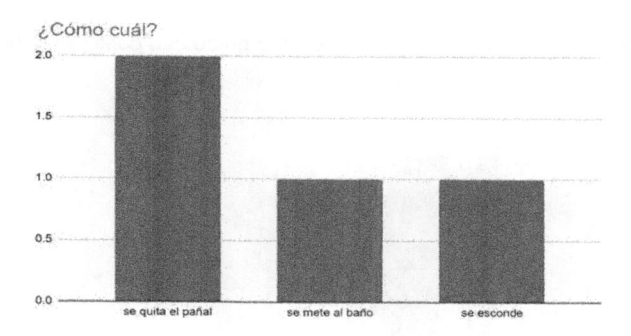

(Bar chart: se quita el pañal = 2.0; se mete al baño = 1.0; se esconde = 1.0)

Some characteristics of the child when he starts is that he begins to know that the diaper is no longer a crucial part of his routine, rather he begins to throw it away or dislikes having it on, as well as asks for privacy to use for his needs.

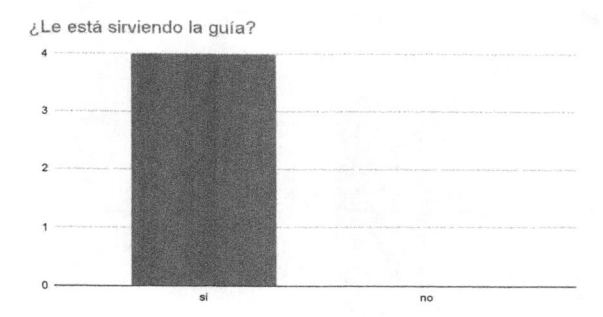

¿Le está sirviendo la guía?

(Bar chart: si = 4; no = 0)

It is important to know if the shared material is helping them to continue using it or to change tactics; the guide was applied for approximately 2 months, which according to the survey in Appendix A is approximately the time that other children mastered the control.

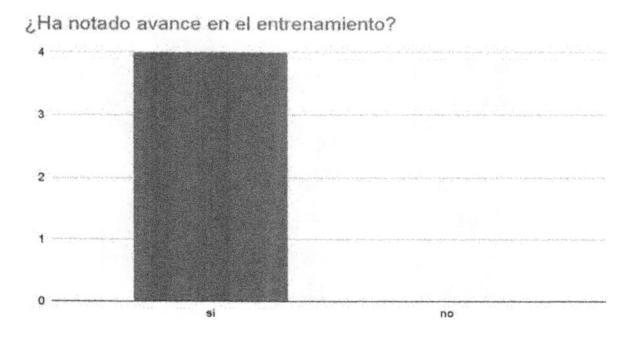

¿Ha notado avance en el entrenamiento?

(Bar chart: si = 4; no = 0)

The child's progress will be crucial to know if the guide can continue to be used as a reference.

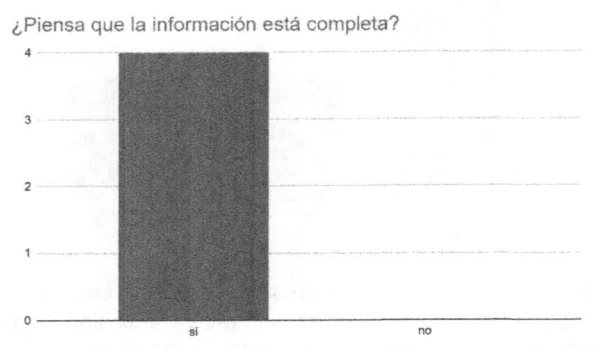

¿Piensa que la información está completa?

Knowing whether the information collected is complete or supportive is highly relevant so that we can change what is not helpful.

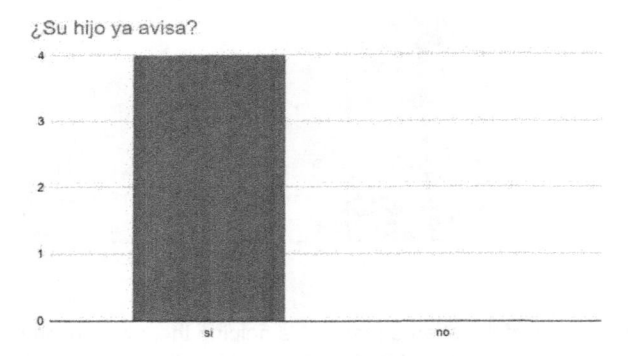

¿Su hijo ya avisa?

The progress that can be seen is important, as it shows how supportive the guidance is being to parents.

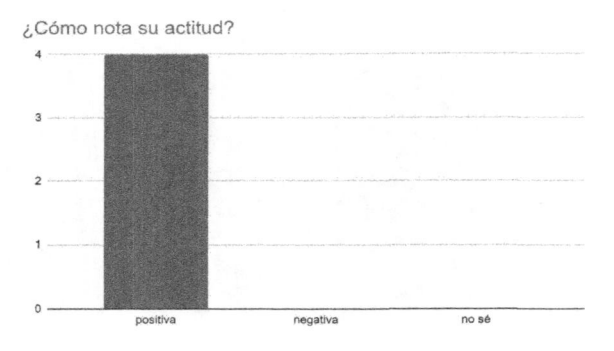

¿Cómo nota su actitud?

It will always be valuable to give the child the importance he/she has, and it will be crucial to know what he/she feels in order to know whether to continue with the training or to postpone it a little, a small advance is better than a big setback in the future.

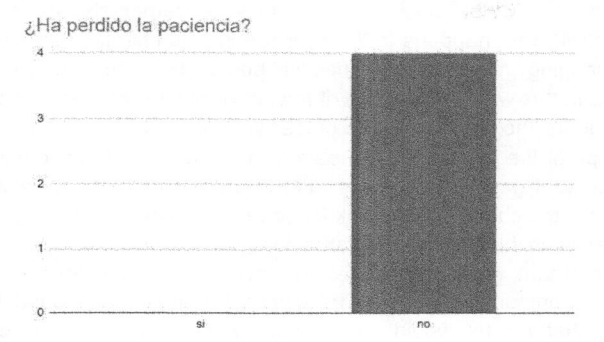

¿Ha perdido la paciencia?

It is also important to know how the parents feel when accompanying their children in the process because when they lose patience, control problems, anger, shouting, insults that often do not want to be said, rather it is what arises from frustration, so it is important to know if the parents are calm. With the answers and testimonies of the parents we were able to confirm that the research, background for the creation of the guide, was crucial to be able to do something that will really help the children, mainly and later on the parents and teachers; knowing about this topic is fundamental, since it occurs in the early childhood stage and is a really valuable aspect for the life of every human being.

CONCLUSIONS

The general objective of this research is the creation of a guide for parents and teachers in the training of sphincter control, taking into account the importance of the child's maturation. At the beginning, we took fundamentals about what is the sphincter control, what happens in the child's body, its changes, its needs, how the types of upbringing influence, the affective bonds, the consequences of the bad accompaniment, this with the purpose of having complete arguments and knowledge about the topic for the creation of the guide.We were able to see that by starting to apply the steps of the guide we were able to provide a good accompaniment to the children because it gave good results, and in a short period of time we could see what happened, the child began to ask for privacy, to sharpen the language, to have more confidence in himself and towards the accompanying adults; to provide an accompaniment that reproves tactics, to have more confidence in himself and towards the accompanying adults. The child felt happier and found the practices appealing so that he/she would begin to have an interest in the subject and to strengthen his/her autonomy.Knowing the maturity needs of children was very important for this research because we understood the characteristics of the stage to start the training, neither before nor after; the consequences of starting earlier, of what could happen if the accompaniment is done in a hurry; knowing what we should do, what we should not do and how to use routines, fun activities, previous knowledge, to achieve one hundred percent control in addition to getting answers from a "saying" of society to have something more truthful and well-founded. This research helped us to know and know what happens in the human body, it is a very important part, because it makes us know what process takes the only sphincter control and helps us to put ourselves in the child's shoes, therefore in the role of support; also made us aware of how the parent and teacher becomes the person in whom the child trusts or will come to do it with the right tools and will do it fully, therefore, we must take care of how the accompaniment is used having that earned trust.It was discovered that this guide could be used as courses or training in childcare centers, since most of the time this is where the child begins with the training, giving more knowledge that can improve the practices of teachers and parents, more than anything else. improve the quality of care given to children so that they can better meet their needs. According to the hypothesis we were able to realize that having a tactical support for parents or companions is of great help, because they had tools on which to base themselves, a foundation to know what is happening in the child's development in addition to respecting the time knowing why children should be given their time to mature.

ANNEXES

ANNEX A

How long did it take for your child to be out of diapers?

How old were you when you started the process?
2 months 2 and a half years
3 months 2 years 6 months
2 months 2 years
Half year 2 years

Do I use a potty or a toilet adapter?

Have you beaten him in his sleep? How many times?
Bacinica Yes 2 times
Adapter Yes, once
Adapter Yes, 4 times
Bacinica Yes, several times

Did you cry in the process?	Did you use a diaper trainer?
No	No
Very little	No
No	No
A little bit	No

In what ways did you support your child? you started?

Did you show interest when

Teaching the use of the toilet Yes to go

Paying attention if he felt like it
Not at first

Paying attention

Yes

Trying to take him whenever he felt the urge to go to the bathroom.
Yes

What do I take into account to start the process?
Diaper discomfort
Teaching you the differences of going to the bathroom Discomfort
Age

ANNEX B

How do you help children with bowel and bladder control?

If it beats it in clothing what do you do?

By not pressuring him and giving him complete security I change it without pointing out that what he did was wrong, but to talk to him so that next time he can warn him.

To help the little ones with potty training I help them with motivation such as a song, stimulating them in a way that does not complicate the process. Reassure the child that it is okay to wet his clothes, that he will do better the next time, that he is growing up and that little by little he will succeed. Taking them to the bathroom constantly, supporting me with songs and stories and congratulating them when they go to the bathroom. Tell him not to worry but to remember to go to the bath so that this accident does not happen again. I support them in their process and congratulate them on their achievements sphincter control has to be with patience and entertainment some games songs that accompany it Change him and encourage him tell him that nothing is wrong and that we will be trying to hug him. First I gain their trust and show them security, then I start to talk to them about what the diaper is, I show them the potty and tell them a little about its function, I invite them to sit down, to explore it, and while they observe it, I tell them that I don't want them to see the diaper and that they can't see it. I explain to him that it was an accident so he doesn't panic and I change it. I tell them to go to the bathroom and every 15 or 20 minutes I help them to sit down so that they build confidence and see that nothing happens, I tell them to go to the bathroom and when they succeed I usually congratulate them and applaud them.

How many children have you helped in the process?
What is your knowledge of the toilet training process?
Very few

Many boys and girls 6-10
Many children since she has been an educator for a long time. 20children That it is a joint process with parents and the teacher. The first thing is that the child is monitored at home for a week with the help of the parents before going to school, then at school he/she will be monitored for 2 weeks. The child should be seated in the cup for no more than 7 minutes. They are stimulated in such a way that the take it easy and motivate the child primarily. They must always have a change of clothes. That if children are forced it can be a traumatic process for them. A basic course of theory for sphincter control but above all the practice is what has taught me that each child has its time to leave it, that we should not force something that are not yet ready because many of the times it is often more difficult for both the educator and the child this process, the child is frustrated by not achieving the goal, sphincter control is certainly a very important issue in which you must give calm and above all dedication because you must be consistent with the procedure and if we do not achieve it. we can cause traumas and problems for the little ones.

What is the method(s) you have used?

Do you use an adapter or potty chair in your job?

Schedule method No,as the bathrooms are suitable for the use of small children.
Songs, a sponge with water in a container to stimulate, representing with puppets in a fun and flashy way. To lose the fear of sphincter control, with lots of motivation like cheers, applause, etc.
Adapter
I don't know the methods, I have only used the one I wrote in the first question.
In employment I have used both but the adapter has worked better for me, because they lose their fear of the toilet.
Games and songs
Adapter

Keeping the potty within reach in one place
Start the process when the child is already well-adjusted in the classroom and I use a potty and only once I applied the adapter but it didn't work very well. with the teacher
Be consistent with the procedure Do not scold or force it.
Celebrate when I make it to the bathroom in the potty.

How long do you leave the child in the toilet?

What recommendation would you give to parents?

5 minutes Fullsupport at home and that there are no reprisals as this would generate a backlash.
7 minutes permaximum That theyhave a lot of patience, that it is a process for children, that they motivate and support them in the process.
Between 5 and 10 min. Thatthe beginning is the most difficult but if they are constant the process will be faster.
Took him every 20 minutes to the bathroom leaving the infant sitting on the toilet in three 5 minutes us more than 7
Patience and, above all, teamwork both at school and at home to carry out the tips given to them and always encourage the child that he/she can do it with support.

I don't have an estimated time, I usually tell them to take their time, there are some children who don't sit for any time at all and there are others who sit for 5 to 7 minutes.

That they be patient with their children, that each one has its own process, some are usually more mature than others and for the same reason some children leave the diaper faster, that they be constant and if they have made the decision to remove the diaper that during the day they do not put it back on, that they do not scold them when they get into their clothes.

Would you like to add more support elements to this area (more adapters, songs, courses, etc.)?

If I consider that as teachers we should receive a course on good sphincter control management
Songs like Pipí sal de tu jardín Popo sal de tu rincón (Several times)

I do not have at the moment.
If all songs games courses all
if the courses for parents, since this process not only depends on the educator but also on a team work with the parents, why not teach them songs to sing to their children, maybe techniques that they can use and implement at home so that the children continue to have this procedure in the best way?

ANNEX C

Does the child show interest in the subject?

Avisa when you've already had a bath?
Can you pull down your pants or underwear?

YES	Yes	No
YES	Yes	Yes
SISi	warns	Yes
YES	Yes	Yes

Does it look uncomfortable when it is done? Does it touch the genitals?

Can you hop with both feet?
Can you follow simple instructions?

Most of the time	No	Yes
Only discomfort	YES	Yes
It is played	YES	Yes
Yes	No	Yes

Awake from a nap?

Can you sit still on the toilet?
Do you show discomfort from the diaper?

Normally	No	YES
Yes	Yes	YES
Yes	Yes	YES
Sometimes	No	YES

Does it empty liquid or are a glass to another with precision

Is there a situation at home that is affecting you, such as: the birth of a sibling, moving house, death of a loved one, divorce of parents?

No	None
YES	None
No	None
No	None

ANNEX D

Is the guide working for you?

Do you begin to see distinct characteristics in the child?

Yes	yes
Yes	yes
Yes	yes
Yes	yes
Yes	yes

How? Have you noticed progress in training?
yes

He asks me to take off his diaper when it is dirty and he starts to feel uncomfortable or tells me he wants to have a bowel movement.

Removes diaper	if
He takes off his diaper and hides for making of the bath	if
He runs to the bathroom and it is his way of notify	if

Do you think the information is complete?

Does your child already warn you?

yes	yes
yes	yes
yes	yes
yes	yes
No	yes

How do you notice his attitude, has he lost his patience?

positive	No
positive	No
positive	No
positive	No
positive	No

REFERENCES

Álvarez , A., & Del rio, P. (1990). Learning and development. La teoria de la actividad y la ZDP. Madrid: Alianza Editorial.

American Academy of Pediatrics (February 11, 2009). HealthyChildren.org. Retrieved from https://www.healthychildren.org/English/ages-stages/toddler/toilet-training/Pages/How-t o-Tell-When-Your-Child-is-Ready.aspx.

American Academy of Pediatrics (August 05, 2013). HealthyChildren.org in Spanish. Retrieved fromhttps://www.healthychildren.org/Spanish/ages-stages/baby/diapers-clothing/Paginas/Dia pers-Disposable-or-Cloth.aspx

American Academy of Pediatrics. (November 11, 2015). American Academy of Pediatrics.Retrieved from https://www.healthychildren.org/Spanish/ages-stages/toddler/toilet-training/Paginas/Toil et-Training-Children-with-Special-Needs.aspx

Andersson, A. (March 21, 2015). Neurology INBA . Retrieved from https://neurologiainba.com.ar/que-es-el-equilibrio/

Arias, S. (2013). Psychologically Speaking . Retrieved from http://www.psicologicamentehablando.com/erickson-y-las-8-etapas-del-desarrollo-human o/ Axarquía, C. E. (2020). National institute of educational technologies and teacher training. Retrieved from http://serbal.pntic.mec.es/pcan0012/documentos/ENTRENAMIENTO-PIPI.pdf

Baby sparks (January 21, 2020). Baby sparks. Retrieved from https://babysparks.com/es/2020/01/21/potty-training-regression-what-it-is-and-what-to-d o/Berger, C., Milicic, N., Alcalay, L., & Torretti, A. (2014). Program for Wellbeing and Socioemotional Learning in third and fourth grade students: description and impact evaluation. Revista Latinoamericana, 169-177.

Bezos Saldaña, L., & Escribano Ceruelo, E. (2012). What do sphincter control problems hide? A case report. Revista Pediatríca Atención Primaria, 317- 321.

Bordignon Nelso, A. (2005). Eric Erikson's psychosocial development. The epigenetic diagram of the adult. Revista Lasallista de Investigación, 50-63.

Burutxaga, I., Pérez Testor, C., Ibáñez, M., de Diego, S., Golanó, M., Ballús, E., & Castillo, J. A. (2018). ATTACHMENT AND BONDING: A PROPOSAL FOR CONCEPTUAL DELIMITATION AND DIFFERENTIATION.
Topics in Psychoanalysis, 1- 17.

Calvo, C. (2020). Chile crece contigo. Retrieved from Ptrotección Integral a la infancia: https://www.crececontigo. gob.cl/columna/avisaba-pero-ahora-no-se-no-se-que-le-pasa/ CAMPO TERNERA, L. A. (2009). COGNITIVE AND LANGUAGE DEVELOPMENT CHARACTERISTICS IN PRESCHOOL CHILDREN. Psicogente, 341-351.

Campo Ternera, L. A. (July 2-December 2, 2011). Psychologia. Advances in the discipline.
Characteristics of adaptive development in children from 3 to 7 years of age in the city of Barranquilla, 95- 104. Retrieved from https://www.redalyc.org/pdf/2972/297224105008.pdf

Campos, A. L. (2010). CODAJIC. Retrieved from Confederación de adolescencia y juventud de iberoamerica y el caribe: http://www.codajic.org/node/2008

Cárdenas Herrera, J. K. (2016). Digital Repository of the National University of Loja. Retrieved from https://dspace.unl.edu.ec/jspui/handle/123456789/11138

Carlos , S. (November 08, 2019). Pediatricsandfamily.com. Retrieved from https://pediatriayfamilia.com/crecimiento-desarrollo/etapas-crecimiento-desarrollo-ninos/

Catalán, S. (June 09, 2012). Educating from family. Retrieved from https://educardesdelafamilia.blogspot.com/2012/06/teorias-psicoanaliticas-freud-y-erikso n.html

CAVANNA, M. P. (February 26, 2013). Natural breeding. Retrieved from https://www.crianzanatural.com/art/art44.html

Cerón Rodriguez, M. (July 13, 2010). MY PEDIATRA. Retrieved from http://www.mipediatra.com/infantil/esfinter-control2.htm

Corbin, J. A. (March 31, 2016). Psychology and mind. Retrieved from https://psicologiaymente.com/desarrollo/teoria-apego-padres-hijos

Craig, Hoffman, Kail, Cavavaugh, Morales, Morris,Sararson (2011). CCH academic portal.
Retrieved from Portal académico del CCH: https://portalacademico.cch.unam.mx/repositorio-de-sitios/experimentales/psicologia2/p scll/MD1/MD1-L/stages_development.pdf

Cuídate Plus . (2015). Cognitive development. Cuídate Plus, 1.

CUSMINSKY1, M., LEJARRAGA, H., MERCER, R., MARTELL, M., & FESCINA, R. (1994). MANUAL OF
CHILD GROWTH AND DEVELOPMENT. Washington, D.C.: Pan American Health Organization.

Del Castillo Sánchez, C. A. (2017). César Vallejo university repository. Retrieved fromhttps://repositorio.ucv.edu.pe/bitstream/handle/20.500.12692/15244/delcastillo_sc.pdf?s equence=1&isAllowed=y

Del Castillo Sánchez, C. A. (2017). Institutional digital repository. Retrieved from Universidad César Vallejo: https://repositorio.ucv.edu.pe/handle/20.500.12692/15244

Del rio, P., & Álvarez, A. (1990). EDUCATION AND DEVELOPMENT: VYGOTSKY'S THEORY AND THE ZONE.

Psychological development and education. II. Psychology of Education, 93-119.

Delgado Ampuero, D., & Zea Vega, M. (2014). ALICIA. Retrieved from Open access to scientific information for innovation: https://alicia.concytec.gob.pe/vufind/Record/UCSM_83d694e3b82f6f7a1506e0921e0f7 83 2.

DELGADO BAZÁN, Y. K., & GARCÍA GIRALDO, Y. L. (2021). Marcelino Champagnat university repository. Retrieved from https://repositorio.umch.edu.pe/handle/UMCH/3228

Dickinson, P. (n.d.). SPHINCTER CONTROL IN. AUTISM99 (pp. 1-10). Badajos: Autism99. Escudero , Á. (2012). The stages of maturational development. Active Training in Pediatrics of.
Primary Care, 65-72.

Faas, A. (2018). PSYCHOLOGY OF CHILDHOOD DEVELOPMENT. Córdoba-Argentina: Editorial Brujas.

Farkas, C., & Rodriguez, K. A. (October 13, 2017). Maternal perception of infant socioemotional development: relationshipwith infant temperament and maternal sensitivity. Acta of Psychological Research, pp. 2735- 2746.

United Nations Children's Fund (1986). UNESCO. Retrieved from UNESDOC digital library: https://unesdoc.unesco.org/ark:/48223/pf0000069549_spa

Font, P. (2015). Institute for the Study of Sexuality and Couples. Retrieved from https://centrodesarrollopsicologico.com/f2018-2020/wp-content/uploads/2018/12/Desarr ollo_psicosexual.pdf.

Belén Foundation (2022). Belén Foundation. Retrieved from https://fundacionbelen.org/taller-padres/etapas-del-desarrollo-cognitivo-cero-tres-anos/

QUERER Foundation (January 26, 2017). QUERER Foundation. Retrieved from https://www. fundacionquerer.org/control-s-sphincters-children-specials-clock-time-potty-watch/

Gago , J. (2014). Open University Program for Older Adults. Retrieved from https://adultosmayores.unr.edu.ar/wp-content/uploads/2020/05/Teor%C3%ADa-del-apeg o.-El-v%C3%ADnculo.-J.-Gago-2014.pdf.

García Ruiz, M. D. (2014). Strategies to address sphincter control in children with tea. Revista digital innovación y experiencias educativas, 1-11.

Garza Elizondo, R. (2020). Sphincter control. Acta Pediátrica de México, 40-42.

GONZÁLEZ ZEPEDA, A. (2004). Contributions of behavioral psychology to education. Revista Electrónica Sinéctica, 15-22.

González, C. M., & Sáenz, C. N. (2020). Respectful parenting: Towards child-centered parenting. Estudios Journal, 1-23.

Guerri, M. (May 1, 2021). PsicoActiva Psychology, testing and Intelligent leisure.

Retrieved from https://www.psicoactiva.com/blog/las-8-edades-del-hombre-la-teoria-del-desarrollo-psico social-erik-erikson/#:~:text=la%20relaci%20relaci%C3%B3n%20maternal.,Etapa%202%3A%20Autonom%C3%ADa%20vs%20Verg%C3%BCenza%20y%20Duda%20(18%20meses%2D,le%20lleva%20a%20the%20verg%C

Guerri, M. (May 1, 2021). PsicoActiva Psychology, test and Intelligent leisure. Retrieved from https://www.psicoactiva.com/blog/la-enuresis-causas-y-tratamiento/

Guerri, M. (May 01, 2021). PsicoActiva.com. Retrieved from https://www.psicoactiva.com/blog/la-teoria-del-desarrollo-psicosocial-erik-erikson/

Guiraldes, E., Novillo, D., & Silva, P. (2005). Encopresis in the pediatric patient. Revista chilena de pediatría, 75-83.

Heras Sevilla, D., Cepa Serrano, A., & Lara Ortega, F. (2016). EMOTIONAL DEVELOPMENT IN CHILDHOOD. A STUDY ON THE EMOTIONAL COMPETENCIES OF BOYS AND GIRLS. INFAD Journal of Psychology, 67-74.

Irurtia, M. J. (2018). Ecuador documents. Retrieved from https://fdocuments.ec/document/trastornos-de-control-de-esfinteres-mj-irur-control-de-e sfinteres-una.html?page=2

Isaza Merchán, L. (2018). CODAJIC. Retrieved from Confederación de adolescencia y juventud de iberoamerica y el caribe: http://www.codajic.org/node/4227

Ketchum, D. (November 20, 2021). eHOW in English. Retrieved from https://www.ehowenespanol.com/las-etapas-del-control-de-esfinteres-de-erikson_126889 46/

Lendoiro, G. (July 15, 2013). ABC parents and children. Retrieved from. https://www.abc.es/familia-padres-hijos/20130713/abci-operacion-panal-verano-2013071 21141.html

López, M. (November 23, 2021). Your educator. Retrieved from https://tueducadora.com/blog/esfinteres/retroceso-control-de-esfinteres#Cuando_se_da_ el_retroceso_en_el_retroceso_en_el_control_de_esfinteres.

Loredo, F. G. (September 02, 2016). Sphincter control. El sol de Mexico, pp. https://www.elsoldemexico.com.mx/doble-via/salud/Control-de-esfinteres-192246.html.

Mansilla, M. E. (2000). STAGES OF HUMAN DEVELOPMENT. Journal of Research in Psychology, 106-116.

Mantilla, M. J. (2019). Bodies, childhood and parenting: bodily cartographies of childhood in the model of respectful parenting in Argentina. Revista uruguaya antropología etnografía, 61-75.

Marchant Orrego, T., Milicic Muller, N., & Álamos Valenzuela, P. (2013). Impact on children of a socio-emotional development program in two vulnerable schools in Chile. Revista Iberoamericana de Evaluación Educativa, 167- 186.

Meece, J. (2001). Child and adolescent development. Mexico City: McGraw-Hill Interamericana.

Mestre , M. V., Samper, P., Tur, A., & Díez, I. (2001). Parenting styles and prosocial development of children. Journal of General Psychology and Application, 691- 703.

Moneta C., M. E. (2014). Attachment and loss: rediscovering John Bowlby. Chiena journal of pediatrics, 265- 268.

Montedonico, F. (2020). Chile crece contigo. Retrieved from Protección integral a la infancia: https://www.crececontigo. gob.cl/columna/crianza-respetuosa-control-de-esfinter/

Muñoz, B. (2022). Montessorizate. Retrieved from https://montessorizate.es/

Navarrete, I., Capano Bosch , Á., González Tornaría, M. d., Navarrete, I., & Mels, C. (2018). From physical punishment to positive parenting. Review of parental support programs. Revista de Psicología, 124-138.

Nuñez Romo, O. (August 2004). Universidad Pedagogica Nacional. Retrieved from https://upnmorelos.edu.mx/assets/desarrollo_fisico_motor_salud_nutricion_1a_inf.pdf

Olivar, T., & Miranda, M. (2013). Physiological changes. THE PHARMACIST, 36- 40.

PACALLA CASTRO, J. P. (2017). Repositori Digital Instituto Superior Japón. Obtenido de http://190.57.147.202:90/xmlui/handle/123456789/1701

Pacheco García, M. T. (2011). THE CONTROL OF SPINTERING IN CHILDREN FROM 3 TO 6.
digital for teaching professionals, 1-7.

Palacios Hernando, C. (June 22, 2022). Making family. Retrieved from https://www.hacerfamilia.com/bebes/quitar-panal-control-esfinteres-panal-20170530142 331.html

Patrizi, E., & Juanico, J. (May 21, 2021). TRUMPET BEHAVIORAL HEALTH. Retrieved from ADVOCACY DENVER: https://www.advocacydenver.org/webinar-control-de-esfinteres-para-personas-con-discap acities/

Pérez Olvera, M. (2006). Adolescent Development III. Mexico: Antología de lecturas .

Pérez Padilla, M. d., Olmos Ríos, F., & Solorio Núñez, M. T. (2019). Socioemotional development in Mexican children: a narrative study on the. PICUMEX, 75-94.

Pinta, S., Pozo, M., Yépez, E., Cabascango, K., & Pillajo, A. (2019). EARLY CHILDHOOD: RELATIONAL STUDY OF PARENTING STYLES AND DEVELOPMENT OF EMOTIONAL COMPETENCIES.
CienciAmerica, 1-18.

Puente, F. (2003). The social maturity of children and adolescents. Educational information network, 1-4.

Quinteros, C., Mariela, E., Elias, V., & Sumiko, F. (2021). Social maturity in early childhood education children of a national and private educational institution, Chiclayo, August - December. 2017. Dspace repository, 1-49.

Rafael Linares, A. (2009). Cognitive development: Piaget and Vigotsky's theories. Retrieved from Universidad Autonoma de Barcelona: https://www.academia.edu/23094319/MASTER_EN_PAIDOPSIQUIATRIA_Desarrollo _Cogni tivo_Las_Teor%C3%ADas_de_Piaget_y_de_Vygotsky

Ramírez Merchán , M. Z., & Rivera Reyes, G. C. (2015). University of Guayaquil Repository.
Retrieved from http://repositorio.ug.edu.ec/handle/redug/14363

Regader, B. (May 29, 2015). Psychology and Mind. Retrieved from https://psicologiaymente.com/desarrollo/teoria-del-desarrollo-psicosocial-erikson

Rivera, N. (March 09, 2008). Gabinete Psicológico. Retrieved from http://gabinetepsicologicobarcelona.blogspot.com/2012/02/apego-vinculos-afectivos-y.ht ml

Robles Bell, M. A., & Basso Abad, R. (2008). Sphincter control training in people with intellectual disabilities. Spanish Journal on Intellectual Disability, 80-87.

Rodrigo López , M. J. (2015). Child welfare and protection. Retrieved from https://www.bienestaryproteccioninfantil.es/fuentes1.asp?sec=25&subs=468&cod=307 1& page=

Rojas , J., Jiménez , C., Mora, A., & Calzada, A. (1999). Scielo. Retrieved from https://www.scielo.sa.cr/scielo.php?pid=S1409-00901999000300004&script=sci_arttext

Shenot , P. (April 2020). MERCK MANUAL. Retrieved from https://www.merckmanuals.com/es-us/professional/trastornos-urogenitales/trastornos-d e-la-micci%C3%B3n/general-about-the-micci%C3%B3n-process

STATE SYSTEM FOR THE INTEGRAL DEVELOPMENT OF THE FAMILY DIF. (2020). Dif tabasco.
Retrieved from http://dif.tabasco.gob.mx/sites/all/files/DIF%20Cuadernillo%20Crianza%20Positiva.pdf

Stanford Children's Health (2022). Lucile Packard Children's Health. Retrieved from https://www.stanfordchildrens.org/es/topic/default?id=toilet-training-90-P05409

UNAM. (2020). UNAM Foundation. Retrieved from https://www. fundacionunam.org.mx/unam-al-dia/la-unam-te-explica-que-es-la-plasticidad
-neuronal/

UNICEF. (2017). UNICEF for every child. Retrieved from https://www.unicef.org/es/desarrollo-de-la-primera-infancia

National Pedagogical University - Hidalgo (2020). National Pedagogical University. Retrieved from Unidad 117, Morelos: https://upnmorelos.edu.mx/assets/procesos-evolutivos.pdf

Urizar Uribe, M. (2012). Basque association of primary care pediatrics . Retrieved from http://www.avpap.org/documentos/bilbao2012/DesarrolloAfectivoAVPap.pdf

Urman , J. (December 12, 2012). IntraMed. Retrieved from https://www.intramed.net/contenidover.asp?contenidoid=16291

Velásquez Cushcagua, A. K. (2018). Digital repository instituto superior japan. Obtenido de http://190.57.147.202:90/jspui/handle/123456789/1838

INDEX

CHAPTER 1 4

CHAPTER 2 16

CHAPTER 3 29

CHAPTER 4 42

CONCLUSIONS 58

ANNEXES 59

REFERENCES 64

More Books!

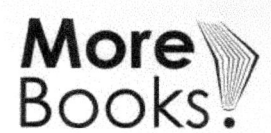

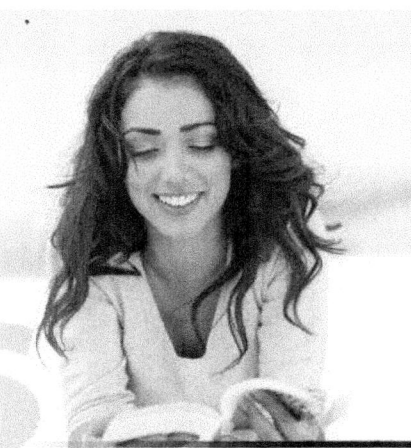

I want morebooks!

Buy your books fast and straightforward online - at one of world's fastest growing online book stores! Environmentally sound due to Print-on-Demand technologies.

Buy your books online at
www.morebooks.shop

Kaufen Sie Ihre Bücher schnell und unkompliziert online – auf einer der am schnellsten wachsenden Buchhandelsplattformen weltweit! Dank Print-On-Demand umwelt- und ressourcenschonend produziert.

Bücher schneller online kaufen
www.morebooks.shop

KS OmniScriptum Publishing
Brivibas gatve 197
LV-1039 Riga, Latvia
Telefax: +371 686 204 55

info@omniscriptum.com
www.omniscriptum.com

OMNIScriptum

Printed by Books on Demand GmbH, Norderstedt / Germany